Gout and coping with gout.

Gout recipes, gout symptoms, purines, causes, remedies, diet, treatments, diagnosis, foods to avoid and foods that might help all included.

by

Robert Rymore

Published by IMB Publishing 2013

Table of Contents

Foreword

When most people think about gout, the only image that comes to mind is that of a limping old man with a crutch and a foot that is heavily wrapped with bandages. This image is a popular one from Victorian dramas and movies set in the era, but the truth of the matter is that gout is a complex condition that affects all types of people.

The American College of Rheumatology reported in 2011 that more than 8 million people in the United States alone were diagnosed with gout. They further reported that the large majority of people affected by gout were men. Going by their figures, about 6% of men in the United States have gout, compared to 2% of women.

These numbers mean that gout is something that you or someone in your family might deal with. Perhaps you know someone who has gout and you want a better understanding of it, or you are in a high-risk group for the condition. Alternatively, you may have recently been diagnosed with the condition yourself and you might wonder what this means to you.

While gout is a serious disease that can affect your life, it is also a condition that can be managed. While no guide can substitute for real medical care, you will find that educating yourself on the condition can go a long way towards empowering you with regards to your own body and your own health.

Learn more about gout so that you can be sure that you are making the right decisions about your body!

Chapter 1) What Is Gout?

Gout is a condition that may seem quite frightening at first. It is easy to get carried away with images that you might half-remember from television shows, movies, and novels, or you may shut down in the face of large amounts of information. If you or someone that you love has been diagnosed with gout, the first thing to remember is that you should take a deep breath. It's hard to concentrate when you are hearing terms like "purines," "gout diet plan" and "remedies for gout" flying around your head, but if you are willing to slow down and start from the beginning, you will feel a lot more comfortable.

1) Definition

At the most basic level, gout is a type of arthritis. It involves an inflammation of the joint that flares up suddenly, resulting in pain, swelling, heat in the area, and tenderness after the swelling goes down. It is a condition that is caused by the build up of uric acid in the blood.

As the uric acid builds up, it forms crystals in the fluid of the joints. These urate crystals can suddenly cause the surrounding area to flare up, which leads to the inflammation and pain of a gout attack.

At the most basic level, gout is caused by the level of uric acid in the blood. There are many conditions that result in irregular levels of uric acid in the blood, and if you are diagnosed with gout, it is important to figure out which ones might be contributing to your issue.

Some of the issues that cause gout can have severe consequences, and after gout is diagnosed, a full physical is often recommended to make sure that the gout is not merely a symptom of a more serious disorder.

Gout is typically a disease that affects the feet, though it can technically attack any joint in the body. By far the most common place to get gout is in the feet, and the most common part of the foot attacked is the big toe. The prevalence of gout in the big toe is such that there is a separate name for the disorder, which is podagra. However, gout is also commonly found in the foot, the ankle, and in the other toes as well.

Gout

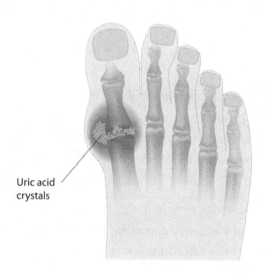

Uric acid
crystals

It is important to remember that there is no cure for gout. If any one says that they have a cure for gout, they are lying to you.

Gout is a condition that you have your entire life. However, the thing to remember is that it can be treated, and it can be managed. It will affect your life, but you can control it to a certain extent. Every case is different, and it is essential to find a set of solutions that works for you!

2) Symptoms

Gout is a condition that is often first noticed when you experience an attack. An attack of gout is characterized by pain that builds up in the affected joint, followed by inflammation.

The joint becomes hot to the touch, and in many cases, it becomes so sensitive that you cannot stand to touch it or put weight on it. In some cases, the pain is severe enough that you cannot even put a blanket on it.

The pain swells and subsides over a period of 5 to 7 days, and in many cases, it is followed by a long period of tenderness in the area.

3) Do I Have Gout?

It always takes a medical professional to make the call on whether you have a certain condition or not. With gout, it can be very tricky because there are a number of reasons as to why you might have an inflamed or swollen joint.

One issue that can prevent the proper diagnosis of gout is that it is a disease that can go quiet for quite some time. Most people notice gout when it is in the acute stage, that is, when they are having flare ups. These flare-ups can occur at any point, but especially at the beginning, there can be lengthy amounts of time when there are no symptoms at all. Some people go as long as 2 years or more between attacks of gout, and this is something that can make diagnosis hard.

If you have recently experienced an issue where you had pain through a joint that was very intense, seemed to have no cause and then subsided again, it is worth having the issue looked over by a physician.

Remember that pain is never normal, and that if you have some, even if it goes away again, you should consider having it looked at.

Do not simply begin treatment for gout without confirmation that this is a condition that you are experiencing. Some of the techniques described here will indeed bring about pain relief, but it is always important to find out about the underlying issue of a condition before you begin treatment.

The last thing that you want to do is to simply treat the symptom of a type of disorder rather than the disorder itself!

4) How Will This Change My Life?

When you receive the diagnosis of gout, you may feel as if your life is whirling around you. Gout is a chronic condition, and if you have never dealt with something like it before, it is very easy to feel as if you and your life have changed forever. It can be tough to get your mind around it, especially if you have always been relatively healthy.

There are definitely a few things that will change when you realize that you have gout and that you need to take care of it, but remember that thousands of people live with gout as a fact of their day-to-day life.

Your diet is likely to be the biggest change that you will need to consider. A great deal of this book is focused on helping you deal with the changes to your diet. After all, eating is a very important part of the way that we deal with our friends, our family and with comforting ourselves.

However, remember that unless you have a very severe case of gout, diet modification is more important than a diet change. In many cases, you will be able to keep your favorite foods, though you may be eating substantially less of them than you were before.

Your doctor might suggest that you lose weight. Gout is a condition that is associated with weight gain. Exercise, when conducted safely and with a clear idea of what is being accomplished, can be very good for a number of things, including lifting your spirits. This is a lifestyle change that might take some time to incorporate, but it is something that can help you to move forward with many goals.

You will need to be more aware of your surroundings and of what is going on in your body. Some people find that they can feel when a gout attack is coming on, and they can take steps to take care of it. This requires you to be more aware of your body and what is happening with it. A greater awareness is also something that can make it much easier for you to figure out what is going on and which foods affect the way that you cope with gout attacks.

Gout attacks involve pain. The pain can be very intense, and it can leave you feeling drawn and exhausted for days. Some people liken the pain to childbirth in terms of intensity. A gout attack can last from days to weeks, but this is something that varies for everyone.

You will need to learn to manage the pain, and you will also need to learn to manage it in a way that keeps you as comfortable as possible.

You will also find that you need to learn how to explain gout to your friends and family. Despite how truly common this issue is, it is still one that is fairly uknown in general. Famous people have had it, but most people associate it with an antiquated time. Be ready to give a quick explanation if you are asked, but also remember that your business is your own. You are the one who decides how much you want to disclose about your own health and wellness.

Depending on the severity of the gout attacks, you may be off your feet for a while. This is something to prepare for in terms of both your job and your social life.

The truth is that after a while, it will simply become normal. Gout is not a fatal condition, and it is not one that will overwhelm your life. The more you learn about it, the better off you will be.

Chapter 2) History of Gout

Gout is often called a modern disease, in that a modern lifestyle in its length and its food choices make it more likely to occur than in the past.

However, it is worth noticing that gout is a condition that has been with us for thousands of years, and in the writings from previous eras, we have discovered that there are plenty of people who fell prey to its pain.

Learning more about the history of gout and some of the people who were affected by it can help you to recognize that this is an illness that does not ruin your life. In fact, some of our brightest minds have dealt with this disorder.

1) Gout Throughout The Ages

Gout is a disorder that has been with people for thousands of years, and the first time that it was mentioned was by the ancient Egyptians around 2600 BCE. There have been mummies unearthed from this era that show signs of gout on the bones of their feet and their ankles. The effects of gout are iconic enough and dramatic enough that they were always noted in various medical reports and histories of the day.

Hippocrates, the father of ancient medicine, further noted the effects of gout many years after the Egyptians. In 500 BCE, he commented on the effects of a condition that he called "the unwalkable disease."

During the medieval period, people thought that health was ruled by the four humors in the body, that is, four fluids that were found in each human body. These fluids were black bile, yellow bile, blood, and phlegm, and it was thought that a healthy person had

13

all of these fluids, known as humors, in balance with one another. It was believed by the doctors and the scholars of the day that gout was a condition that occurred when one of those humors would drip into the joint in question. The term gout itself comes from this belief, as it is derived from the Latin term, *gutta*, meaning drop.

Though the mechanics behind gout were not easily understood, it was evident even to people in past times that there were some factors that seemed to be part and parcel of gout. For example, during the Victorian period, it was known as a rich man's disease. It was only the rich that could afford the vices that were known to be associated with gout.

Given the fact that gout has always been such a dramatic and obvious condition, it makes sense that people throughout history were concerned about gout causes and gout remedies. They wanted to know what causes gout, and there were a variety of things used as gout medication.

Because the symptoms of gout were so obvious, it became a simple thing for people to identify gout, but learning how to treat it effectively was another story.

As little as a hundred years ago, gout was a disease that could render someone completely unable to walk. Even now, when it is not treated correctly, gout symptoms can make life very difficult. However, we are long past the point where we believe that it is solely rich food and alcohol that causes this condition.

Gout was also a condition that people sought to cure in various ways. In the Victorian era, bed rest and hot bandages were typically prescribed; with the hot bandages bringing relief to the pain and ideally some reduction of the swelling. In the days of Byzantium, some 2000 years ago, physicians were using derivatives from the autumn crocus plant in order to reduce the pain. It is interesting to note that the autumn crocus plant contains colchicine, an alkaloid that has proven effective in issues related to swelling and inflammation.

Gout is an interesting disease in history specifically because of its place among the affluent. For example, the Romans have detailed records of an aristocracy that suffered intensely from the effects of gout; something went with the rich wines that they drank and the extremely rich food that they ate. Similarly, the Victorians believed that the disease itself was something that only rich people acquired. One lord famously called gout the disease of the gentleman, differentiating it from rheumatism, which he decried as the disease of the coachman. In form if not in accuracy, that lore was correct. While both gout and rheumatism are types of arthritis, they are each caused by different things.

2) Famous People With Gout

Sometimes, when you or someone you love has a condition like gout, it is worth knowing that you are not suffering alone. There are many people who have gout today, and although the disease is now more common than it was before, there have been many famous people throughout history who have had it.

One of the most famous gout sufferers in the United States is Benjamin Franklin, famed for his understanding of electricity and his contribution to the Declaration of Independence. In fact, during the drafting of the Declaration of Independence, he suffered from a gout attack that was so intense, he could not attend the meetings. Instead, he had to have the drafts delivered to his home so that he could look them over.

Franklin was a man who definitely considered things like herbal remedies for gout and gout home treatments. At the time, there was no real understanding of the anti-gout diet, and gout treatment at home was largely what was available.

However, Franklin seemed to have a thorough understanding of what not to eat when you have gout. In a display of his trademark wit, he wrote "Dialogue Between Franklin and the Gout," where he gives his gout the personality of a strict lady. The piece is dated Midnight, 22 October 1780, and anyone who has ever suffered a gout attack can sympathize with Franklin's writing. In it, he implores the gout for relief, while the gout scolds him for being too fond of rich food, too little interested in exercise, and forever making excuses as to why he will not be healthier. In the end, he calls her tiresome, but recants quickly when she threatens another visit. The piece ends with gout stating that she is his friend, though whether Franklin believes her is left unstated.

Some scholars believe that gout has changed the course of world history at least once. King Charles I of Spain was a monarch who controlled a fair part of the world in the 16th century. By the age of 16, he was appointed the ruler of Spain, a position that put him in control of vast holdings throughout Europe, North America, and South America. By 1528, however, Charles began to show signs of gout, which was at the time often called the disease of kings.

Though he was crowned the Holy Roman Emperor not much later, Charles was unable to push the boundaries of his vast kingdom any further due to his condition. His gout attacks became so bad that he needed to postpone commanding his army to take Metz, a city in Flanders. Charles, who had been an active military leader in his youth, eventually needed to abdicate his throne in favor of his son Phillip II. Charles was a ruler who was known for his empire and his ambition, and if his rule hadn't been curtailed relatively quickly, the Spanish Empire could have gone to be even more prolific and extensive.

Another kingly sufferer of gout was King Henry VIII of England, who is perhaps most famous for having six wives throughout his life. Though the most memorable picture of King Henry is one that shows him at his heaviest in his middle years, the young King Henry was quite athletic and handsome, an active man and a romantic king.

However, in 1536, King Henry took a bad fall in a jousting accident. This lead to a thigh injury that never quite healed right, instead becoming sore and ulcerated. This, in turn, prevented Henry from being as active as he would have preferred to be. Due to inactivity and depression, King Henry put on a great deal of weight, and this, in combination with a rich diet that only a king of the realm could afford, lead to issues and complications with gout, which further reduced his mobility and his ability to live in a healthy way.

Gout is also a disease that can attack people who are otherwise healthy. For example, one modern gout sufferer is the actor Jared Leto. While working on the film *Chapter 27*, where he played Mark David Chapman; the man who shot Lennon, he was asked to put on weight to better suit the character. The relatively slender Leto went on a regimen of melted ice cream mixed with soy sauce and olive oil to put on weight, a routine he stated was much more difficult than losing weight. This resulted in an impressive weight gain of more than 60 pounds, and though Leto was able to do the movie, it lead to him acquiring gout.

The sudden weight gain affected Leto's body in a dramatic way, and the actor reported pain and inflammation that was so severe, he had to use a wheelchair. This is just one example of how gout can occur in the modern era, even when the causes are understood.

There are many people who have suffered from gout in the past, and there are more being diagnosed every day. Though gout is something that does impact your life, you will find that it does not need to be something that consumes you.

Chapter 3) Who Gets Gout?

The question of who gets gout is one that often troubles people. Though we now know that the causes of gout are more complex than what people have previously thought, it is worth understanding what your risk factor might be. You may know all about how home remedies for gout treatment can work, and you might be up to date on the best gout flare-up treatment, but do you know what is causing you all of the pain? Learning more about who gets gout can help you to determine where your risk behaviors are. You can learn to skip certain foods to avoid gout, and progress with your treatment in peace.

1) Alcohol Use

Alcohol use is thought to increase the risk of gout due to the fact that beer specifically has a high purine content. Purine is a substance that needs to be broken down in the body, and when it is broken down, one of the byproducts is uric acid. In a normal system, the uric acid leaves the body through urination, but in some cases, the kidneys are unable to process the uric acid. It stays in the blood and eventually transforms into the urate crystals that attach themselves to the joints and cause gout.

A study published in the Lancet Medical Journal showed that when a population of 47,000 people with no history of gout were followed for 12 years, 2 percent of the men involved had some issues with gout over that time. From that group, individuals who drank alcohol on a daily basis had twice the risk of developing gout compared to people who did not drink. Each glass of beer per day increased the risk by about 50 percent, while drinking hard liquor only increased the risk by 15 percent.

Though there are plenty of natural gout treatments out there, it is far better to simply avoid gout as a disease if at all possible. Think about your drinking habits and consider how they might be affecting your body's ability to function well. A little bit of thought can go a long way, and if you are a beer drinker, particularly if you are a male drinker, it may be worth your while to consider whether you should cut back. When it comes to gout, natural treatments are great, but in general, it is far better if you can avoid the entire mess!

2) Foods High in Purine

In the past, gout was called the disease of kings and the rich man's ailment. What this tells us is that rich foods have always been associated with gout, and that typically means red meat, among other dishes. Purines are found in food just as they are found in alcohol, and because purines are typically not harmful unless you actually have gout, it might not be something that you have ever considered. Thanks to diets and other health issues, you may know which foods contain fats, carbohydrates and sugars, but do you know what contains purines?

All meats contain purines, though there are some that are particular offenders. Oily fish like tuna and salmon are high in purines, as are scallops and lobster. Red meat is high in protein, and some of the types of meat that are the highest in this substance are livers and kidneys. Comparatively, chicken is lower in purine, but it might still be a risk factor.

Some vegetables are also considered high in purines. Lentils and beans of various types are rich in purines and should be limited. Similarly, cauliflower, spinach and asparagus are all foods to be approached with caution. Mushrooms of all sorts can also be problematic.

Finally, yeasts are known to be sources of protein. This is

especially notable in beer, which uses yeast in the fermentation process, but it is also worth noting that this can take some breads and probiotic foods out of your diet as well.

It is important to remember that eating these foods does not guarantee that you will get gout. There are plenty of people who eat these foods and never have any issues at all. However, if you are someone who comes from a family with issues with gout or if you are concerned that you have already had a gout attack, it is in your best interests to control the amount of purines that you put in your body.

3) Gout and Weight

The relationship between gout and weight is one that is somewhat tricky. There are definitely large people who do not have gout, and there are definitely thin people who do, but according to the study mentioned above, there does seem to be a correlation between weight and gout.

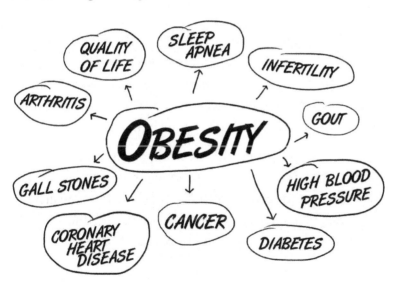

Men from the study who were overweight or who put on weight

over the time period were more likely to get gout than men who were not. Alternatively, men who lost weight managed to reduce their chances of getting gout by around 40 percent. This weight loss was only calculated to about 10 pounds, that is to say, only a loss of 10 pounds correlated to the loss of weight. More weight lost would not necessarily convert into to a lesser chance of developing gout.

However, also be aware that, when you are looking at gout and what causes it, losing weight suddenly or putting it on quickly seems to have more to do with gout than being heavy your entire life. The truth seems to be that the body simply does not like rapid changes of any sort. Crash dieting can definitely contribute to strange responses in the body, and rapid weight loss, especially when the person in question is dealing with a lot of yo-yo dieting, is something that can induce gout. Be aware of this before you attempt any sort of weight loss in the future! A sudden drop in weight can also stress your body to the point where it has a gout attack.

It does seem clear that reducing weight can mitigate the factors that cause gout, but it is important to remember that the weight loss may be incidental. Most standard diets recommend cutting back on foods that are high in purine, like red meat, and cutting back on these foods does correspond to weight loss.

Remember that crash dieting will not work, and as you look over things like symptoms of gout in feet and natural treatment for gout, it is important to remember to direct your efforts towards the right place. Gout signs and symptoms are varied, and remember that correlation does not imply causation.

4) Gender

When it comes to groups that commonly get gout, men are high on that list. One explanation for this discrepancy is that at puberty, the levels of uric acid in the blood of men rises sharply in contrast to the levels found in women of the same age.

This results in between 5 and 8 percent of men developing uric acid levels that put them into the hyperuriecemia category, where they are prone to developing gout. However, it is also worth noting that it often takes between 20 to 40 years of this condition before a gout attack occurs. Men tend to develop gout somewhere between the ages of 30 and 50.

Women, on the other hand, tend to have significantly lower chances of getting gout until after they have gone through the menopause. Though the mechanism is not entirely understood, it is thought that estrogen plays a part in preventing the rise of uric acid in the blood. When it comes to women who suffer from gout, only 15 percent of this population manifests a gout attack before the onset of menopause.

By the age of 60 or so, the likelihood of men and women developing gout is about equal.

5) Gout and Heredity

As with most disorders, it is worth realizing that there is a genetic component to gout. If people in your family have gout or have had at least one gout attack, it means that you are in a group that is considered at risk. About 20 percent of men studied who have developed gout know of at least one family member who has the disease.

If you have a family member who has gout, it is worth your while to be careful about the condition, to take care to eat well, and to be very careful about the purines that you introduce to your diet.

Be aware of your family history, and make sure that you speak to the people that you need to. Talk to older family members before you lose your chance, and talk to more distant family members before you forget about it. Even if they do not tell you anything useful for yourself, you may find that they can help your own immediate family.

Just because someone in your family develops gout does not mean that you suddenly need to start looking up gout diet recipes or a gout diet sheet. Simply be aware of the issues and take a moment to consider what a gout diagnosis could mean to you.

If you have a family member who deals with gout attacks on a regular basis, consider yourself lucky that you have a resource. Ask them what food to avoid for gout, and consider what gout treatment guidelines they follow. While the condition is different for everyone, you will find that the way that they feel about gout and diet can help you to understand your own situation a little bit better.

6) Gout and Medications

There is a strong correlation between gout and some medications. Basically, any medication that is known as a diuretic is something that can concentrate purines in the blood and lead to a gout attack. Diuretics are prescribed for a number of different ailments, among them, high blood pressure. Diuretics are very commonly added to drug regimens, so be aware that if you have gout attacks, it might be time to talk to your doctor about what your diuretics are doing and whether you should stop them or find a replacement. Cyclosporin is a drug that is most frequently given to patients who have recently had an organ transplant. It works by decreasing the patient's immune system to the point where it does not resist the new organ or attack it. However, thanks to the immune system suppression, it can make people prone to gout attacks that were not so vulnerable before. As a matter of fact, any drug that suppresses the immune system can make it difficult to fight off gout, so keep this in mind if you are looking to mitigate the causes.

Some painkillers or drugs used in painkillers can cause gout attacks. Salicylate is a common additive to over the counter painkillers, and although they are used to treat gout pain, they can also interfere with the kidney's function. Kidney function is a primary part of how the body fights off gout attacks, and once that function starts to waver, the gout attacks can occur once again.

If you are worried that the medication that you are taking puts you at risk of gout attacks or you are concerned that your medication is making your existing gout attacks worse, talk to your doctor at once.

The medication that you take is a serious thing, and if you are really being affected by the drugs you are taking, no amount of careful eating and exercise is going to get you where you need to be. The fact that gout attacks are so influenced by medication means that you need to be very aware of what is going into your body and what you can do about it.

6) The Unknown Factors

Sometimes, people with no history of gout and absolutely none of the other risk factors end up with gout. The thing to remember about gout is that it is an illness. It is not something that you bring on yourself, and it is not something that you have any control over.

Part of the thing that makes dealing with gout such a problem is that people feel guilty about it. They think that they could have prevented it with a better diet, or more exercise or less crash dieting.

They might also think that they have lost control over their own lives or that now that they have this issue that they are no longer healthy. The important thing to remember is that your gout is a condition. It affects your life, and it can definitely make some things very hard, but the truth is that it does not change who you are.

There is no reason to feel guilty about having gout, any more than you should feel guilty about tripping and spraining your ankle.

Look at your gout as a problem to be solved, not a judgment or a punishment, and you will have a much better course towards recovery and treatment.

Chapter 4) Gout Diagnosis

As we mentioned before, gout is something that cannot be diagnosed simply by looking at the symptoms. What looks like gout may be a simple injury or an infection or any number of other things. If you are worried about gout affecting your life, you need to take yourself to a doctor to learn more about how you should proceed.

You cannot form a treatment plan until you have a diagnosis, but if you are like many people and afraid of the unknown, the doctor's office can be more than a little frightening!

Quell some of that nervousness by making sure that you know what is going to happen if the doctor needs to talk to you about gout. Gout is not something that can be diagnosed by simple observation. There are three tests that might be used to diagnose the presence of gout in your body.

1) Joint Fluid Test

A joint fluid test looks for urate crystals in your joint fluid. This substance is a thick liquid that is found inside the joint itself. Its purpose is to lubricate the joint and to make sure that it can move easily. When urate crystals are observed in the joint fluid, it is often assumed that gout is the culprit.

A joint fluid test is slightly uncomfortable, but it is conducted over the space of just a few minutes. Depending on your doctor and your situation, you might be given a local anesthetic to the area beforehand.

If you are worried about a needle going into your body, look away from it. The professional administering the test will have no problem completing the test as long as you stay relatively still.

This is a very common test, and there is no reason for you to stay at the hospital overnight or to worry about being kept.

After the joint fluid is drawn, you might find that you are slightly tender and sore in the area. Typically, all you need to do is to chill the area with an ice pack to remove the pain from the procedure.

2) Blood Test

Though joint fluid is the preferred medium to search for urate acids, there are a few things that might prevent the fluid from being taken. For example, if you are currently suffering from a joint inflammation, it might be difficult to get a needle into the joint appropriately. Similarly, if your insurance will cover a blood test but not a joint fluid test, you may end up with a blood test instead.

Blood tests are less accurate when it comes to actually defining the possibility of gout. These tests are designed to detect high levels of uric acid in your blood. Uric acid can point to gout, but there are also plenty of people who suffer from high levels of uric acid who never have to deal with gout at all.

Essentially, a blood test is often used as a confirmation of gout if you have already had an attack, or it might be used as a warning sign if you have never had gout before. Some doctors will see a high level of uric acid as a good reason to put you on a low-purine diet.

When you get a blood test, the procedure is relatively simple and straightforward. You will be sent from the doctor's examining room to a place where a phlebotomist works. He or she will sit you down, and use an alcohol swab to clean off the area at your inner elbow. They might lightly thump your skin to bring veins to the surface, making them bigger and easier to locate. This is where the skin is very thin and where you can easily have a needle inserted without too much trauma.

The needle used is very thin, and though there is a sharp prick when it goes in, there is usually no pain after that. The blood is drawn very quickly, and depending on the tests that are used, the phlebotomist might draw one to three vials of blood.

Afterwards, the needle is withdrawn, and the area is swabbed with a cotton ball and bandaged. You can leave the bandage on for twenty to forty minutes, after which, you can remove it entirely. There may be a slight bruise, but there should be no blood at all.

3) Urine Test

The third way to test for gout is to go in for a urine test. This is the least popular way to test for gout, but increased levels of uric acid can be found in urine, just like it can be found in blood.

A urine test is usually done immediately at the hospital, but if you cannot produce a sample at the time, you may be sent home with a sterile container and then asked to bring the sample back to the lab. Typically, there is no appointment needed to drop off a medical sample.

Chapter 5) Gout Treatments

When you are thinking about uric acid gout remedies and other things, you may be less inclined to worry about things like what purines are than you are to be concerned about man-made and natural gout remedies. The good thing about gout is that there is plenty of information out there. After you are done asking yourself what the symptoms of gout are and you have an idea of the foods to avoid for gout it is time to look at what remedies you might consider.

1) NSAIDs

Next to learning what foods to avoid when you have arthritis conditions like gout, one important thing for you to be aware of is the use of NSAIDs. NSAID stands for non-steroidal anti-inflammatory drug, and they are designed to bring down inflammation and bring relief to the body. They are typically used as painkillers, and they are also useful when it comes to bringing down fevers.

At higher levels, NSAIDs are used to bring down swelling, which is where they are often brought in when it comes to gout. While there are plenty of great gout natural remedies out there, you may find that your best friend is going to be an NSAID that you can buy over the counter or one that is prescribed to you by your physician.

The important thing to remember is that gout is a condition that is very persistent, and that the inflammation that is suffered by people with gout is a symptom of the issue, not the issue itself. When you take an NSAID for your gout attack, you are not fighting the gout; you are simply making the pain easier to bear.

Gout is not something that you cure with NSAIDs.

That being said, there are several types of NSAIDs that are typically used for gout attacks. First and most commonly, you will find that ibuprofen is recommended as a quick fix. This is available at your local drug store, and it can be purchased quickly and easily, though it is worth your while to talk to your doctor if you end up taking it regularly. Ibuprofen can have long-lasting effects on your body if it is taken regularly for an extended amount of time.

Some other NSAIDs that might be prescribed to you include diclofenac, indometacin, sulindac, and naproxen. These NSAIDs are fairly strong, and they all need to be taken exactly as the directions state. Do not take more than is prescribed, no matter how bad your pain might get. If you have issues with your NSAIDs, speak to your doctor right away. While some people search for a perfect home remedy for gout, and others look for food to avoid with gout or foods to avoid with arthritis, you can begin your campaign against gout pain with a very simple pill taken as needed.

When it comes to arthritis, natural remedies are very helpful, but don't be afraid to supplement them with NSAIDs. NSAIDs are very useful when it comes to pain relief and pain management, so consider adding them to your natural arthritis remedies today. Natural gout treatment often does best when it is coupled with medication of one sort or another.

2) Probenecid

When the key is to prevent a gout attack rather than to reduce the effects of one that is progress, one drug that you might be prescribed is probenecid. This drug is used almost exclusively to treat gout and arthritis with gout like tendencies, and it is from a family of drugs known as uricosurics. Probenecid is a drug that reduces the amount of uric acid in the body as well as helping the body to get rid of the uric acid that is already there. It is also often used in conjunction with penicillin, because it reduces the kidneys' ability to remove the drugs from your system.

When probenecid is being used to combat the effects of gout, it is typically taken twice a day, orally. It is considered best to make sure that this medication is taken with food in the body to prevent rejection and nausea, and it is also recommended that the medication be taken with a full glass of water.

Although probenecid is taken to prevent gout, it does nothing for a severe gout attack, and it can even make a gout attack worse if it is taken at the wrong time. After the medication is begun, gout attacks might substantially worsen for a short time, but after that, they typically dip significantly. Speak to your primary care physician about what you can do to reduce issues while you are on probenecid, especially if you feel that your gout attacks are not subsiding quickly enough. This is a medication that performs best when it is taken regularly, so be sure that you take it as recommended by the doctor.

It is also important to be aware that probenecid is not considered a pain reliever. If you do have a gout attack, drugs like ibuprofen should still be taken to combat the pain.

3) Colchine

Colchine is an alkaloid drug that is frequently used to treat gout both when you are having a gout attack and also when gout attacks need to be prevented.

In a higher dose, it is designed to mitigate the effects of a gout attack. It is often the first medication that is used when doctors are trying to help you get through your first gout attack, though it is important to remember that colchine is not without its side effects. Firstly, it can make eating difficult, as the dose used during attacks is frequently associated with nausea. It can also be linked to diarrhea, which can make an already difficult situation even more uncomfortable. Depending on the situation, the nausea and the diarrhea may indicate that the drug should be replaced with another medication, but that is between you and your medical professional.

After the first gout attack has subsided, it is typically prescribed in a much lower dosage, where the side effects are reduced, if not non-existent.

When colchine is a medication that is being considered for either gout attacks or as a preventative measure, it is important to have a complete physical history presented to your doctor. There are a number of conditions that make a person unsuited for long-term use of this medication. For example, if you have recurrent kidney problems, heart problems, or gastrointestinal problems, you will find that this medication is not suited for you.

Fortunately, for most people the effects of colchine are mild. While you are taking colchine, it is very important to make sure that you are staying in contact with your health care professional. They should be monitoring your health and testing your blood yearly, just to make sure that this drug is not creating a problem elsewhere.

4) Corticosteroids

Corticosteriods are a family of drugs that use steroid hormones to reduce swelling, among other things. These medications are prescribed when NSAIDs are not enough or when they have become ineffective at controlling the pain and the swelling from a gout attack. They are also typically the medication that is used when colchine is ruled out of a person's treatment. Corticosteroids are medications that may be administered in pill form, or they may be injected directly into your joint, which is slightly more painful. Doctors are often willing to give corticosteroids on the same visit when you need to be tested for gout in order to provide a quicker relief.

Though they are a fairly safe medication for gout, it is still important to remember that corticosteroids are not without their risks. When taken over an extended period of time, they can inhibit healing wounds, and they can also reduce your ability to fight off illness. One long-term possible side effect is thinning of the bones.

Typically, it is recommended that, if you need to use corticosteroids, you receive the lowest dose possible, and that you remain on them for the shortest amount of time. Many doctors prefer to offer corticosteroids as a drug designed for quick relief. They can work wonders when you are suffering through a gout attack, but after they have done their job, you will be recommended a different drug to take on a preventative basis.

5) Xanthine Oxidase Inhibitors

When you need to look into drugs that actually prevent the occurrence of a gout attack, you will find that the first choice is frequently the family of drugs known as xanthine oxidase inhibitors. These drugs lower the levels of uric acid in your blood, and there are a number of different options available.

Allopurinol is one of the most common generic drugs offered for gout attacks, but it is important to remember that it comes with a risk of low blood counts and rashes. Febuxostat, on the other hand, may come with nausea, a rash and reduced liver function.

When considering these drugs, it is essential that a gout attack be completely resolved before xanthine oxidase inhibitors are started. It has been found that if these drugs are taken before the attack is completely resolved, it can actually lead to a new, severe attack. One way to prevent a second attack from occurring is to make sure that someone is started on a low dose of colchine and then transitioned to the xanthine oxidase inhibitors in a few weeks.

6) Pain Management

A big part of dealing with gout is not necessarily about preventing an attack, but in dealing with an attack when it shows up. Gout attacks are painful, and they can leave your joints feeling so tender that you cannot even cope with having the pressure of a sheet on them.

The first line of defense that is generally recommended is over the counter medications like ibuprofen and aspirin. However, it is important to remember that aspirin especially can take a toll on your body, with particular focus on your kidneys and your liver.

Consult your doctor if you are taking over the counter medications on what is turning out to be a regular basis. They may want you to limit your use, to try another over the counter medication or to move you to a prescription painkiller.

Pain management is a tricky thing, and it is different for just about everyone. Only you can tell how bad your pain is; do not let anyone tell you that it hurts less or more than you know it does. If you are honest about your pain, you are taking the first step towards ensuring that you get the right kind of treatment for it.

Pain management can take many forms, many of which are discussed in the section "Coping With Gout."

One important aspect of pain management is that you need to be aware of your body and your surroundings. Gout is a chronic issue, and once you have it, it will always need to be something that you think about.

Be willing to make allowances for yourself. If you feel that a food or an activity is going to activate your gout attacks or make them worse, take the time to find a way to work around it. Be willing to talk about your needs to the people around you, and consider what alternatives might exist.

A big part of pain management is simply being willing to say that you are in pain, and that you need to find a solution. Do not assume that your pain will go away if you ignore it, and do not think that simply because you get through today that you will be able to do so tomorrow.

Pain is your body's way of telling you what is wrong, so respect it!

Chapter 6) Coping With Gout

If you or someone that you care about has been diagnosed with gout, it can feel as if your world is shifting. You have been diagnosed with a possibly debilitating disease that will give you a severe amount of paint. You may feel as if your life is shifting out of control or that there is nothing that you can do.

While it is true that gout is a chronic condition, you must remember that you are not helpless. There is plenty of information out there when you are looking for a diet for gout, for home remedies for gout or for foods that cause gout.

Even if you are already receiving plenty of medical help and advice, you will always be ahead of the game if you are willing to be proactive about your care. Looking up gout home remedies, gout diets and what gout is caused by is something that can help you feel empowered. Whether you want to know more about gout causes and symptoms or you are on the hunt for a gout natural treatment that works for you, start your search today!

1) Gout Journaling

When it comes to looking at gout diet restrictions and trying to find the best gout treatment for you, it is very easy to start to get confused. You may be wondering whether that last natural gout remedy that you tried was really effective, or whether symptoms of the gout treatment you last tried were different than they were before.

As with any medical issue, keeping track of things like your day-to-day health and the medications and herbal gout remedies that you were considering can be difficult. There is a lot to remember, and remedies for gout pain can be quite diverse. As you proceed, you may find that there is no perfect remedy for gout pain, but instead you can create a perfect solution for your own needs.

As the doctors keep telling us, every person is different. No matter what you see on commercials, there is no one-size-fits-all solution when it comes to a problem like gout. Gout affects people in different ways and with different types of severity, and you never know when a solution is going to work for you.

With this in mind, a health journal is something that can be very helpful for you. A health journal is something that you can use to keep track of the gout symptoms and treatment plans that you have tried, a particular food to avoid, or the gout home remedy that you were considering. As you may have noticed, gout food to be avoided by one person is food that can be easily eaten by another.

To make a journal that you can carry around with you, simply pick a notebook from the store and clip a pen to it. Date the page, and write down anything that is pertinent to your condition. Some people take their notes in a very free-form way, while others prefer to answer the same questions over and over again.

For example, a list of questions for your gout health journal might include:

* Am I suffering from gout pain today?

* If I am suffering from gout pain, what is its intensity? (You may choose to rate the intensity of the pain from 1 to 10, just to give yourself an idea of whether the pain is increasing or decreasing over a certain span of time.

* What have I eaten today?

* Am I on my period?

*How much water have I drunk today?

*What medications have I taken today?

*What was my level of physical activity today?

These questions are just designed to get you started. You can answer them as completely and as detailed a fashion as you like. You are creating a record for your own use, though you may find that it is helpful to refer to this record when you are dealing with your doctor as well.

You may also find that there are apps for your Smartphone that will help you to keep track. There are several apps that tell you how much purine is in the food that you eat, and there are many general health apps out there that will tell you how much you have eaten in general and how healthy you are on a given day.

Apps tend to be a little less precise than keeping track of your condition on your own, however, so consider keeping a few notes of your own.

While keeping a journal might feel a little demanding or tedious at first, you will quickly find that in no time at all, it can make a huge difference to how you are looking at your health.

A big reason to try the gout journal is to simply remark on your food. Because many of us are so busy, it is often a lot of trouble to think about what we eat. We run to the fast food place around the corner, or we don't think about the snacks that we are currently consuming.

A food journal forces you to record everything that you eat, and if you know that you need to make the entry, you might find yourself pausing to think.

On top of that, a good health journal will also ensure that you record what treatments you have started and when they began. For example, a journal will help you figure out when you started the type of medication or when you began a treatment. In many cases, the treatments that you began will only begin to take effect slowly. Without a clear idea of when you began them, you might begin to grow impatient when it really takes several weeks to work, or you might continue a treatment that doesn't work for you believing that it will take more time.

A gout journal can go a long way towards teaching you more about how you are doing. It makes you stop to reflect what is going on with your body, and it makes you much more aware of how you feel.

Remember that a gout journal can be whatever it needs to be. While plenty of people prefer to have it in a physical form that they can carry around with them, other people prefer it to be an app that they fill out on their tablet or their Smartphone. Others prefer a middle of the road approach where they type all of their data into a document on their computer. If you decide to type your information into a document, consider getting a cloud-based archival service, so you have access to your document no matter what machine you happen to be on.

2) Be Patient

Remember that any treatment or diet that you use to treat gout should not have instant results. Even NSAIDs, which work to bring down inflammation and swelling, can take some time to work to their full efficiency.

Nothing is fixed overnight, and as with any other individualistic problem, you will discover that it might take you some time to get where you need to be.

Do not be discouraged when you are dealing with yet another gout attack. It can be painful to remember that this is a chronic condition, but the truth is that you will see some improvement with some diligent effort. You may feel as if you are helpless in the face of the pain, but the truth is that you do have some power over it.

It might take you weeks or even months to get a really good grip on what works for you, but once you have it, you will be in a much better place.

One of the worst things about the first few gout attacks is that you do not know what is going on. You are in a great deal of pain, and you may feel afraid as to what is going on in your body. This can make your situation seem even worse.

3) Support

When people think about treatment for gout, they often think solely in terms of methods to relieve pain. Given the fact that pain is such a significant part of this disorder, that makes sense, but there is an entire mental and emotional side to the disorder that needs to be addressed.

For example, you may feel that you brought the disorder on yourself. You may be ashamed of choices that you have made in the past or you may be worried as to what others think of you. It is essential to remember that gout is a disorder like any other. There is no one thing that causes it, and in many cases, it is often a perfect storm of attributes that bring it around.

Alternatively, you may be upset at the loss of mobility. If you are an active person, gout can put a serious kink in your plans. Depending on what you did before you suffered from gout, you may feel as if this condition has robbed you of important parts of your identity.

A diagnosis of gout can spin your life around. It is a chronic disorder, and it can affect you in many different ways. Do not be afraid to be sad, upset, or angry about it, and do not allow anyone to tell you how you should feel. While you should of course control your actions, you are entitled to feel how you want to feel about something that changes your life.

Look for support when you need it. Take advantage of your family and friends, and take them up on their offers. In many cases, it is too easy to feel as if you are a burden when the truth is that most of your friends would love to sit and hear about your remedy for gout or to find out what gout is caused by. They want to listen to you, they love you, and they care about you, so do not shut them out.

Be ready to give a little bit of education about gout as well. After all, gout is a bit obscure when it comes to portrayals in the media, and your friends will not know what foods cause gout or the signs and symptoms of arthritis pain. They will not know what foods to avoid with gout, which can make going over to a friend's place for a meal a little tricky, and they won't know about purines in food, all things that you have had to become an expert on.

Be willing to be an educator and to make sure that they know where you stand. Tell them about home remedies for gout pain or the brand new natural remedy for gout that you are currently invested in. A little bit of education can go a long way towards getting your friends to be the support group they want to be, so be willing to share with them and to help them understand where you are coming from.

4) Rest

One of the things that they do not often tell you about pain management is that pain is tiring. Even when you are not actively in pain, even when the pain itself is something that you can consider minor, you may find that you are simply tired all the time.

Firstly, think about why this is true. Gout causes pain that radiates from your joint to the rest of your body. That means that your body tenses in reaction to this pain. Constant tension throughout your frame is something that can leave you feeling exhausted!

When you are always tensed up, it does not matter what you know about foods causing gout or what causes gout. All that matters is that pain is radiating through your joint, causing your whole body to tense. The gout in foot symptoms that you might be suffering from are causing your body to stiffen up, and hold itself tense, and that is why a good gout remedy treatment will always include some kind of pain management.

Even when you are eating well and aware of what foods to avoid for gout, you will discover that you are getting tired. A gout attack makes your muscles tense up tightly, and when this happens, you will find yourself stressed out and exhausted.

Make sure that you account for this pain when you are having a rough time. If you feel a gout attack coming on, or you are recovering from one, you should remember that you are going to be tired. This means that you should be prepared to spend some time recuperating.

If at all possible, go to bed early. It is usually better to go to bed early and to wake up at your normal time rather than to simply stay up late and sleep in. This keeps your circadian rhythm on track, and it prevents you from staying up late when you are recovered.

Some people have a rough time sleeping if they are in pain, so consult your doctor about things like painkillers and sleep aids that are designed to be taken right before bed. Some people like to use medication to help them get to sleep, while others prefer to rely on natural methods, like warm almond milk and meditation.

If you want to take a natural approach to getting to sleep, the best thing that you can do is to create a wind-down routine. Half an hour before you actually go to bed to sleep, turn down the lights. Take a warm shower so that you are feeling relaxed, and consider eating something relatively light but full of protein.

Keep the room as quiet as you can, and simply let your mind drift. If you want to read before you to go sleep, do it in a chair rather than in the bed. If you can make sure that the bed is associated only with sleeping, you will be able to drift off much easier.

Before you go to sleep, take off your watch. Some people find that they are constantly checking the time as they sleep. They are either worried that they have to be up too soon, or they are concerned with how little sleep that they are getting. If any of this is the case for you, remove the watch, triple check your alarm if you need to, and put away this distraction.

Remember that sleep is when your body has time to heal from the problems that have been affecting it through the day. If your gout pain is preventing you from sleeping, it will only get worse. Some people manage to reduce their sleep until they are forced to fall asleep and then to build up to a full's night of rest in a short while, but this is something that can take time and effort.

When you are looking up herbal remedies to help you with sleep, consider valerian and St. John's wort, though you should check with your doctor to make sure that you are not getting anything that will interfere with your medication.

Another natural option for you to try is melatonin, which is often called the sleep hormone. Melatonin is a hormone that your body produces naturally, and it is what is used to send you to sleep. In many cases, the human body does not produce enough melatonin, and beyond that, disrupted lives and pain can reduce the production of melatonin even further. Pick up a bottle of melatonin at your local vitamin store, take it about half an hour before you mean to go to bed and see how well it works for you.

Remember that if you lose enough sleep, you can be as impaired as if you were drinking! Too little sleep takes a slow and gradual toll on you, and over time, it is something that will decrease your quality of life. Your mood starts to slip long before you think it does, your functionality goes way down, and you will discover that in no time at all, you are letting things slip that should not slip.

All of these symptoms are very serious, so when you are worried about them, or you are afraid they are affecting you, call your doctor.

If you are having pain on your foot, consider what you can do to keep your foot still. Some people pile up blankets on either side of the foot, creating a hollow. When your foot is placed in this hollow, it becomes much less inclined to roll around. If your foot is sensitive, stabilizing it can help you sleep through the night.

Remember to be gentle with yourself when you are looking at recovering from a gout attack. This is a paint that some have compared to childbirth, and you will discover that it can leave you feeling exhausted. Get the rest you need, and you will be on your feet much more quickly than you might be if you had pushed yourself.

5) Water and Plenty of It!

We're told over and over again that water is good for gout, but what you might not know is why.

At the most basic level, water washes waste material out of your body. It allows your body to get rid of waste products from various metabolic functions, and it allows you to make sure that you do not have that waste causing harm in your body. You've heard the standard idea that everyone needs to drink at least eight glasses of water every day, but the truth of the matter is that in general, the more water you drink the better!

When you drink enough water, you are creating a way for your body to get rid of such things as the uric acid, which builds up and causes the crystals to form in your blood. When you keep your system well hydrated, you are creating a situation where you are keeping your uric acid levels as low as possible.

While some people do just fine when they are told to drink more water, it can be a little troublesome for people who never drank all that much water in the first place. As a matter of fact, most of us go through our lives being vaguely dehydrated without ever even knowing it!

How can you make sure that you get the water that you need? The right amount of water for you is a personal thing. You might choose to stick with the common eight glasses of water a day rule, because that will tend to get more water into you than not, but if you have a little more time, it is worth listening to the new scientific wisdom.

According to scientists today, to get the best use out of the water that you drink, take your body weight in pounds and divide that number in half. That number, in ounces, is how much water you should drink.

Take a moment to think about when and where you get your water. Some people drink their water with meals, but for the best results, you should consider drinking your water about an hour before you eat. This prevents the food from soaking up the water and carrying it out of your system before you can take advantage of it.

Consider getting a drink of water part of your daily routine. Get up and drink a glass of water, and then make sure that you have a tall glass whenever you take a break during the day. On top of that, consider having a glass of water a little bit after you work out or a few hours before lunch.

When you are thinking about how you can move forward towards drinking more water, consider carrying a water bottle around with you. A water bottle is a constant reminder that you should be drinking more, and if you want to make the water more interesting, you can add a little bit of flavoring, like with a squirt of lemon juice.

Remember that the best thing to drink is pure water. While things like sodas and teas are quite tasty, they are also diuretics. They encourage the water to leave your system sooner than it should, and with regards to gout, that is the last thing that you want.

Try to drink water whenever it is offered. When you are at a restaurant, ask for water, and when you pass a water fountain, take a drink. There are many great benefits for getting more water in your system anyway, so take the time to make sure that you are taking care of this basic gout attack preventative.

One important note to remember is that if you are taking any medication for your kidneys or if you are on any kind of diuretic, as people often are for their high blood pressure, contact your doctor about how much water you should be drinking.

6) Reduce Stress

Many people note that stress is something that brings on a gout attack. Sometimes, it is stress over work, and other times, it is stress over a family member or a romantic entanglement, but one moment, the person is frustrated about something, and in the next moment, they are dealing with sharp pains in their feet! Stress is something that can weaken your body's immune system and prevent it from fighting off gout attacks as effectively as it should. Stress is something that can take almost any situation and make it worse, and when you are dealing with something that comes and goes like a gout attack, you will find that it is time to see what kind of stressors you can remove from your life.

When it comes to how to treat gout, there is just so much information out there. Between natural remedies for arthritis, learning about purine foods and considering a uric acid diet, it can be hard to stay cheerful. As you contemplate a low purine diet and inform your family about your diet restrictions, you may start to feel a little run down.

This is exactly the kind of environment that can make stress much worse, and when you are looking to keep yourself healthy, that's when stress can attack.

At the most basic level, stress is a fight or flight experience. It is designed to help us fight off attacks from people who would do us harm, and it can also make sure that we get away if we decide to run. However, stress and adrenaline, the chemical that enables us to do these things, do not have the same applications as they once did. We can no longer run away from a fraught meeting with a family member, and we cannot simply punch a customer who is being annoying, even if we wish we could.

Instead, the stress builds up and builds up, and if we don't let it out, it starts to manifest in unhealthy ways. Some side effects of stress include panic attacks, anxiety, hives, constant fatigue and short tempers. In the case of gout, stress can actually induce a gout attack.

When you first look at it, calming down the stress in your life feels like a huge task. Often, most of the things that are stressing you out do not have easy answers. If they did, you wouldn't be stressed out about them! However, you will find that it is essential for you to both identify the type of stress you are experiencing and then to figure out how to calm your reaction to it.

When you are trying to identify the source of your stress, think about when you feel the most frustrated or the most helpless. Too many people think that there must only be one thing that is causing them stress, when the truth of the matter is that it is likely to be several different things.

Think about what you feel throughout the day. Sometimes, the thing that is causing you stress is such an every-day occurrence that it startles you to realize that you are harboring such frustrated emotions so often.

If you are feeling stumped when it comes to sources of your stress, start keeping a journal and note down your feelings throughout the day. One way to organize this is to divide the page into two columns. Label the column on the left "Things That Happened," and label the column on the right "How I Felt." If you start to fill this out truthfully, you will soon discover the source of your stress.

Once you have figured out why you are feeling stressed, you need to think about what to do. Stress is an emotion that leaves you feeling tired and drained, but it is not because you have done something. Instead, it is frequently because you were not able to do something.

One saying goes that you should control what you can control, and do your best to work around the rest. If you are constantly pounding your head against something that cannot be changed, you are not going to feel better. Accept that some things are beyond your power and move on. Although you might fear that this is too much like giving up, the truth is that it simply means that you are preserving your energy for a better purpose.

Create a plan of action. If you are someone who thrives with lists and rules, you will quickly discover that they can make you feel better about things that are stressing you out. Think about the problems that are frustrating you at this moment, and think about what you can do about them.

If there are things that you cannot change, you should find out how you can make it so that they do not bother you so much. For example, if you have a family member who is behaving poorly, think about a way to make sure that you stay away from them until they improve or the circumstances change.

There are many methods that are ideal for making sure that stress leaves your body, and many of them are great for gout as well. Check the section below for exercise and how to do it in a way that will not hurt you, but also consider things that will smooth away some of the ragged edges of the day. You may know all about low purine recipes, gout diet plans and gout symptoms treatment, but do you also know how to take care of yourself.

When you are just getting used to the symptoms for gout and learning what gout symptoms are, you may have forgotten about some of the things that usually relax you. If reading that made you think that it's been a while since you've watched a movie or did some knitting, pick it up again. Our brains love patterns and even if you are suffering from gout symptoms, you can enjoy them. Meditation is a great choice for getting stress relief from gout, and though you might associate it with highly spiritual people, it is in fact an exercise that you can use in your day-to-day life to center yourself. Meditation can last anywhere from a few minutes to a few hours, and when you are getting started, look for meditation tracks on streaming sites like YouTube. Get the track started, and simply meditate as long as it takes to finish the track.

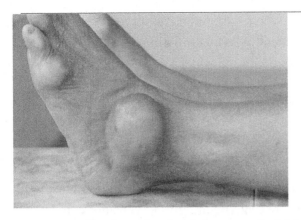

To start meditating, simply sit in a comfortable way that will not allow you to fall asleep. Let your eyes drift shut, and concentrate on your breathing. When you first start meditating, thoughts will drift in and out. Let your mind think about them, but do not dwell on them. Think of your mind as a river or a stream. Focus on one segment, and just as things come in, let them drift away.

Empty your mind, slow your breathing, and for the length of the track, just exist. You have many things going on in your life, not in the least of which is gout, but for the moment, you do not have to think about them. You are giving yourself a break. You will take up your responsibilities in five, ten, or thirty minutes, but as you exist right now, you do not need to think about anything at all. Meditation is a great way to reduce stress, and in that way, you can use it to prevent gout attacks.

When you are looking for a more active way to relax, you might consider volunteer work. Even if you are working under the assumption that you will have bad days with your gout, and even when you are concerned about what you can really handle, there are some fantastic activities that are perfect for you.

Remember that while gout can take some things away from you, it cannot take away the person that you really are. The issues with gout that you have do not change what your mind and your spirit are like. If you are not worried too much about decreased mobility and you are relatively healthy, why not volunteer with your local park service? If you love kids, consider joining a free day care program, and if you have a knack for computers, offer to do some coding for the local non-profit of your choice!

7) Exercise

Think about starting an exercise regimen that you really love. Exercise creates a situation where stress can leave your body and where you can make sure that you are giving your body the movement that it needs.

Before you start exercise, however, it is important to speak to a doctor. This is especially true if you have not exercised in any sort of concentrated way in the last few years. People like to say that exercise is something that everyone should do, but the truth is that not everyone should do it in the same way. If you have undiagnosed herniated disks, for example, exercise that does not take them into account can actually leave you bedridden and in worse shape than you started out.

If you are overweight, there is a chance that a doctor will okay you for exercise without much of an exam or a talk. This is a sign that the doctor is not seeing beyond your weight, and it is also a sign that you need a new doctor! Exercise creates stress in the body, and if you do not know what you are doing, it can actually create chronic issues that will be with you for years, if not decades. Talk with your doctor about a thorough physical, any physical issues that might have you concerned, and which exercises might be right for you. Someone who is relatively healthy will likely do fine with a heavy cardio workout, while someone with weaker or damaged joints might need to stick to low-impact exercises like water aerobics or yoga.

Remember that exercise is something that needs to suit you. Do not push yourself to do a kind of exercise that frustrates or annoys you. While no pain, no gain is widely dismissed as a poor way to get in shape or treat your body, it cannot be denied that exercise is an investment in time, and often in money.

Think about your life and first consider where exercise can fit in. While it has some great health benefits, the amount of stress that is caused when exercising can be significant. For example, think about whether you want to exercise before or after work, with friends or completely on your own, and how much money you can spend on it. Your exercise needs to fit into your life. It should not be a cause of stress!

Remember that you will miss a workout from time to time. The key is to make sure that you make each missed workout an incident rather than a trend. Plenty of people miss workouts here and there, so do not feel demoralized if you do too.

What kind of exercise appeals to you? When it comes to dealing with gout, nearly any kind will do. A gout attack can leave you unable to workout in some ways, but there are still exercises that you can do to stay limber. During a gout attack, you need to take care of yourself, but otherwise, the rest of the time, exercise can often be conducted normally.

Try to find a type of physical activity that you can look forward to. If you are someone who is deeply interested in time outside, by yourself, think about going for solitary runs in the park. If you love the feeling of camaraderie and you have a performing streak, think about joining a dance troupe. There are plenty of great ways for you to get exercise out there.

If you love zombie movies, pick up a Smartphone app that shows you how to get in shape for the zombie apocalypse, and if you are worried about people seeing you and making fun of you, pick up a jump rope and work out at home.

8) The RICE Method

If you have ever been around people who treat or receive sports injuries, you have likely heard about the RICE method of treating sports injuries. One thing that you may not know, however, is that it is also a great way to treat the affected area before, during, and after gout attacks. While the cause of gout is not always known, and while gout diet foods have changed as our understanding of the condition has gotten better and better, the RICE method, in one form or another, has been used consistently. RICE is an acronym that stands for Rest, Ice, Compress, and Elevate.

Rest is obvious, and when you are looking over a gout diet menu and deliberating between gout treatments, you might not be inclined to do anything but rest, but this can serve as a reminder. Gout attacks take a lot out of you, so as you go over your gout diet list one more time, get some rest.

Ice is used to cool the inflammation around the area and it can also be used to bring down swelling in the affected location. Ice is also used to numb the area, meaning that as you work on your gout symptoms diet, you will be able to reduce the pain as well. Be careful with ice as it is possible to overdo it, but in general, if you wrap the ice in a thin towel, you will be fine. If you do not have ice to hand, you can simply use a frozen television dinner or other frozen boxes to cool your inflammation.

It is important to remember that the use of ice in gout treatment is somewhat controversial. Some people adore the use of ice to treat their gout attacks, while other people shudder to think of the cold on flesh that is that sensitive.

Experiment with it to see how you find it to work for you. You may be able to take some cold, you might love having it on your painful area, or you might not like it at all. It is always worth remembering that every home treatment for gout is different, and what works for someone else might not always work for you.

To compress an area affected by gout, you can use a standard bandage or you can simply do it much more gently with a long towel or length of fabric. One great thing to do is to heat a towel in the microwave and to use it to gently wrap the area. Do not wrap the area too tightly. A tight wrap is intended to help you move around, and if you have a gout attack, you want to avoid that as much as possible. Heat a towel very lightly in the microwave, wrap it around your foot or ankle, and settle in to look over your gout diet list.

Finally, elevate the affected limb. It sounds almost cartoonish, but you can actually drain the blood from the inflamed area by getting gravity on your side. Use a cushion or a pillow to prop your leg up. Some people even do this when they sleep.

The RICE method is definitely something that should be included in your gout self-care regimen, right up there with gout herbal remedies and lists of gout diet foods to avoid.

9) Heat

When it comes to home remedies for gout treatment, heat is one of the things that often gets brought up, but some people find that its use is controversial. They say that heat only makes the area more inflamed and does no good at all. While cold is often recommended to relieve pain, it is important to remember that heat serves a different purpose.

The addition of heat can bring more oxygen to a wound, helping it to heal more quickly. This means that heat is often traded off with cold when it comes to treating gout.

As any gout remedy report will tell you, exercise is important.

However, if you are stiff from a recent gout attack, it is not safe for you to immediately jump into your aerobics program! This is where heat can come in. Use heat to loosen up the affected area before you start your exercise routine, and then afterwards consider icing it to calm down the area. Remember that any really severe gout attack means that you should be very careful with yourself, just as you know to be careful about gout and foods to avoid.

Be very careful with heat, as some people find that its use makes the area worse. Other people enjoy the pain relief that they get from the heat, but find that they need to drink a lot more water to cope with the dehydrating effect of the heat.

Do not use extreme heat of any sort to treat gout; keep it mild.

10) Finding a Herbal Remedy for Gout

When it comes to looking up gout remedies, natural options are sure to come up. As a matter of fact, there are many natural remedies for gout, and herbal options are often milder and less severe in terms of side effects than drugs that you would get over the counter or from the doctor.

As you look up natural treatments for gout, you will find that most of the herbs that are recommended for natural treatment of gout all have a certain factor in common. They are all used to treat inflammation of the joints. Virtually any herb that is commonly used to treat inflammation can be used to treat gout. As you consider your gout treatment, natural remedies can play a big part in how you go about it.

As you look into gout foods, one of the best things that you can do is to look into supplements that are made from foods that are high in anti-oxidants. Anti-oxidants work to remove inflammation from your body, and some of the most effective ones include blueberry, bilberry, rapeseed, and pineapple supplements. Bilberry and pineapple are especially great options to consider when you are looking at gout treatments that are more natural. Bilberry is rich in anthocyanin, which are designed to help your body direct its blood flow. This is an excellent thing in a gout attack, where blood flow is slowed in the affected area. Pineapple supplements are rich in bromelain, a substance that helps the body to reduce the amount of uric acid in the blood.

Another great herbal remedy to try when you are looking at figuring out how to create a good treatment for gout is devil's claw. Devil's claw is a distinctively shaped herb that is also often called the unicorn plan. It is available in a dried, powdered capsule form, making it easy to ingest, and it does several things to help with gout. It is a powerful anti-inflammatory, and it is also thought to lower the levels of uric acid in the body.

This herbal remedy is typically taken when the first twinges of a gout attack start, and people speak enthusiastically about it bringing down the length of a gout attack from weeks down to mere days. When you are looking at gout treatments, natural remedies might be more effective than you thought. Devil's claw is easy to find at any reasonably stocked vitamin or alternative health store, and it is definitely worth a shot.

As you consider your gout treatment, natural methods can show you the way. The right treatment for gout varies from person to person, but as you learn more about the causes of gout, you can also learn a lot about gout home remedies for pain treatment.

11) Accept the Fact that Gout Attacks Will Just Happen

Even people with excellent management techniques and a thorough idea of what they are doing are going to have gout attacks. Remember that gout is a chronic condition and that no matter what you do about it, it will affect your life. No matter how much you know about foods for gout diet, what to eat for gout diet or gout treatment diet home remedies, there are going to be days where you find yourself dealing with gout attacks.

Some people get very demoralized when they feel as though they have done everything right, and they still get gout attacks. The truth is that you can be on the most rigorous purine diet for gout treatment and you can be on great medication for gout treatment, and you might still have an attack.

This does not mean that you should give up all hope of stopping a gout attack! It only means that you are not perfect and that your body simply functions in a way that is less than desirable. Do not fault yourself for something you can't control.

12) Manage Your Pain

If you are aware of the right gout diet for you, and if you are being otherwise very careful, you might start to get a little worried about the pain. You may begin to feel that the pain is your fault, or that you can tough it out.

Pain is not a punishment, it is not something that you need to endure, and whether you bear it quietly or loudly, it comes to the same thing. Pain is simply your body telling you that there is something wrong.

Gout attacks bring pain with them, and as any medical professional will tell you, pain is not a mild thing. It is a serious condition that can make your life very hard. It can stop you from doing things that you want to do, and it can make you feel extremely vulnerable.

Do not think that you have to bear pain in silence. Pain does not get better unless you do something to stop it, so be aware of your pain and advocate for yourself. If your medication is not working to control your pain, talk to your doctor. If a certain type of exercise is aggravating your pain, stop and find an alternative option.

Simply enduring pain silently is something that we are taught is a virtue, but the truth is that it does not serve us well.

If you are in pain, the best thing that you can do is to treat it or find a way to mitigate it.

No one is saying that you should expect the pain to go away entirely. Just be aware that there is a space between no pain at all and searing agony. Do not be afraid to look for pain management solutions.

You get no credit and no gain from staying silent, so speak up!

13) Regular Doctor Visits

If you have a serious case of gout, the truth is that the doctor is going to want to see you on a regular basis. If you were relatively healthy before, you may have managed to skip regular visits routinely.

However, the thing to remember is that knowing what foods you should avoid if you have gout and gout diet causes are just the tip of the iceberg. When it comes to good gout medication, treatment involves getting yourself to a professional.

Remember that the levels of uric acid in your blood should be regularly monitored, and that your doctor is the only one who can perform the tests. Learning what gout foods to eat and avoid is also something that your doctor can help you with.

Speak with your doctor about how often they want to see you. Depending on the case and depending on what your needs are, they may be fine seeing you once a year, but some want to see you every six months or even more often.

One of the best things that you can do when you are looking at staying healthy while dealing with gout is to consult with professionals regularly. They are the ones that can tell you when a change is just a normal thing and when it is something to be seriously worried about, and they can also help you to figure out what you need to change.

Try to make sure that you see going to the doctor as a necessary thing, rather than something that you can just do or avoid as you please!

14) Learning to Say No

One thing that is going to surprise you, especially if you have never had to deal with any sort of eating restriction before, is how pushy people can get about food!

It takes a lot of time and effort for you to figure out what not to eat for gout and to look into food that causes gout, and that's after you've weeded out the pseudo gout diet plans out there that get in the way!

After you've spent all this time gathering the knowledge that will keep you healthy, it is entirely fair for you to get irritable with all the people who say "but just this once won't hurt!" or "you just need to try this steak, it'll be fine!'

Food is one of the ways that we make others feel included, whether we understand that or not, and sometimes, it seems that others do not care about what gout is and the symptoms associated with it, they just want to make sure that you try their liver and onion dish!

Be very firm with people, and remind them gently that you are dealing with a medical disorder. This is not something that they have a right to pressure you over, especially if they are the kind of people who want to push the latest homeopathic gout treatment or pseudo gout treatment onto your lap. If they get aggressive, remember that you have a right to look after your health, and that you are the person in charge of what you put into your mouth!

This is not to say that you will not be tempted. Sometimes, people will just want to go to the sushi place where all you can really have is cucumber roll, and sometimes, you will go to a family dinner where all you can eat are the whole-wheat bread rolls.

This can be a tricky situation to deal with, but one thing that you can do is to pre-eat. Before you go, eat a full meal of something that you have prepared for yourself, and that you know is safe. When you get to the event itself, you can simply eat appetizers or anything else that is safe.

When you are dealing with a trip, do your best to pre-plan. Look over menus for fast food places that will be en route. Places that prepare personalized sandwiches are your best bet for staying safe, as is any place that has a good menu for vegetarian cuisine. If someone else is planning the trip, make sure that they are aware of your needs.

Remember that you should also consider what to do at social drinking situations. Sometimes, it's hard to be denied your favorite drinks when everyone else around you is having a good time. One way to feel a little better about this is to volunteer to be the designated driver. You might also bring up the situation with a close friend and ask if they want to keep it limited with you when your friend group goes out.

Saying no to anything can be tough, especially when people are asking about things that you previously would have been delighted to accept. Remember that you are doing what you are doing for your health, and stick to your guns!

15) Take a Footbath

As you learn more about gout remedies at home and as you reach out to look for the gout cure treatment that will work for you, it might be a good idea to start taking footbaths, or simply learning to submerge any affected part in hot water. Remember that using heat is a bit controversial in the gout community, but there are enough people who get good results from it for you to give it a try!

As you are learning what foods to avoid when you have gout, also think about the kind of home care treatments you can do. A footbath is a simple thing, and when you are dealing with a gout attack, you will find that it can make a huge difference to how you are moving forward.

To take a footbath, you simply need a foot basin from the local drug store. Just about any bucket or container will do, but it is a good idea to make sure that your feet have enough space and enough room so that you can stretch out and feel really comfortable.

Fill the foot basin with enough hot water so that you can completely submerge your feet, and simply sit and soak in the luxury for a little while. You can stay in for just five minutes if you want some instant relief, or you can simply use the footbath for an hour or so, adding warm water as the water cools down.

While you can certainly leave the footbath plain, there are a number of different things you can add into the mix. For example, some people find that adding a few teaspoons of Epsom salts to the water can help reduce swelling and bring about pain relief, while other people swear by adding a few drops of their favorite essential oils, like lavender and citrus.

One of the interesting things about the uric acid crystals that cause gout is that they are soluble in heat. As a matter of fact, it only takes a few degrees above body temperature to make them dissolve somewhat. However, as the body lowers to the normal temperature, they will re-form.

Whether a warm water bath works for you or not is a personal thing. Some people enjoy instant relief from a footbath, while other people find that they do best when they keep the area at a steady room temperature.

If the footbath makes your foot feel worse instead of better, don't do it. Do not use a footbath where the water is simply too hot, and make sure that you dry your feet completely afterwards.

16) Gout and Acupuncture

When you are in a spot where you are interested in making sure that your gout gets better and you would like to try some alternatives to drugs, it is worth your while to try acupuncture. Acupuncture is a method used in Traditional Chinese Medication, and it is shown to have some excellent effects on both reducing the pain of gout attacks and reducing the frequency as well. Acupuncture relies on the insertion of very thin hollow needles into specific points on the back, arms and legs. In some cases, the practitioner might run small jolts of electricity through the needles in order to stimulate the muscles. Though it might look a little alarming, it is generally quite painless. Afterward, people report feeling a great deal more energetic and dealing with a great deal less pain.

When you go looking for an acupuncturist, remember that you can treat it in the same way as when you are looking for a doctor. Find out who is recommended, ask people in the community, and go in for a consultation rather than an appointment.

Talk with your acupuncturist and ask where they studied. If you get any sort of strange vibe from the office, back away and try another clinic. The truth is that, as with so many other decisions to be made about your health, this is all about your comfort level.

You will often need to strip down to your underwear when you are dealing with an acupuncturist, and if you wear a bra, you might be asked to remove it. If this makes you uncomfortable, bring a friend or ask the person performing the procedure if there is anything that they can do to work around it.

When you go in to speak with an acupuncturist, make sure that they know what you are going through and the kind of problems that you are hoping to relieve. There are many people who are interested in acupuncture for a variety of reasons, so be willing to be explicit.

Ask them what you can reasonably expect in terms of improvement, and be diligent in monitoring it for yourself. Some people find that acupuncture works very well for them, and others prefer to stick to their own methods.

Chapter 7) What Food Causes Gout and What Foods Help

At this point, we know that food does not necessarily cause gout. Instead, it is a matter of a number of different factors. However, when it comes to gout, what not to eat is something that comes into play fairly heavily. As you learn what the symptoms of gout are, and gout causes and treatment, you will learn a lot more than you knew before about this condition. Chances are that you will find that there is no one gout cause or any particular symptom of gout for you to look for.

With that in mind, however, it is going to be handy for you to have a list of food categories for you to be careful about and to watch out for. No matter what causes gout in your body, you will find that in general, there are some foods to pay attention to.

1) Meat

All meat contains some purines, but in general, go a little lighter on the meat than you have been. The standard serving of meat, no matter what it is, should be about the size of a deck of playing cards or your palm. That means that you should eat this amount of meat just once a day, ideally.

Do your best to skip meats that are particularly rich. Red meat, duck, and fatty seafood are all high in purine and associated with a lifestyle that is at risk for gout. Skip the tuna, the scallops and the steak to achieve a lower level of uric acid in your blood.

Organ meats are a poor choice for anyone who happens to be on a gout diet, as are any broths that have been cooked extensively in bones and other connective tissue.

One thing that often sneaks up on people is the fact that anchovies are in a fair number of things that are otherwise quite innocuous. For example, anchovies or similar fish are often used in Asian fish sauce, which can make many Asian dishes rather risky. Worcestershire sauce, found in most standard grocery stores, is made through much the same process.

When you are looking for good meat to eat, keep it lean. Mild fish, that is, fish that does not come with a lot of oil in it, is a good choice, as is lean chicken breast.

Basically, the richer a meat is, the more likely it is that it will give you problems. This does not mean that you have to cut meat out of your diet entirely, however. Lean meats and white meats are still perfectly acceptable, and white fish, like tilapia and sole can be just fine if your case of gout is relatively mild.

You will also find that moving your protein consumption from meat to beans and tofu is a great idea. These are low-fat sources of the protein that you need, and they can even help you to defend yourself against gout attacks. Learn how to make some delicious veggie burgers in the recipe section. It is not meat, but it will give you a chewy texture that does very well in your day-to-day cooking. Meat can be a tough thing to reduce in your meals, but just remember that you do not need to remove all of it, and that there are other ways to get the food that you require.

2) Seafood

When it comes to talking about foods that are forbidden on a low purine diet, seafood comes up very quickly. However, the thing to remember is that while you should definitely cut back on your consumption of seafood, you do not need to limit it completely.

Seafood is like every other category where there are some things that are better for you than others.

For example, most crustaceans are straight away out of the question. Lobster and crab are both very high in purines, and they can give you problems right away. However, fake crab, often spelled krab, is typically made out of white fish, which is lower in purines. Do check to make sure that you know what your imitation crab is made up of before you proceed, however.

When it comes to fish that you should be very careful with, at the very top of the list are the oily fish. Herring, tuna, and salmon are all oily fish, and although they contain the extremely healthy omega 3 fatty acids, they are also high in purines. However, there are also milder fish out there that do not trigger the response in people who are less sensitive.

Be careful about eating any kind of shellfish. Oysters, clams and scallops are all high on the list of fish to avoid, even in broths.

Think about the different kinds of seafood that you eat and consider which ones have to leave your diet.

3) Alcohol

Alcohol prevents your body from getting rid of purines, so be willing to cut back. Beer is the biggest culprit, and if you are having a gout attack, skip the beer entirely. It is not known how much beer you can drink before it becomes a problem. White wine, on the other hand, is relatively safe, and a glass a day will not hurt you with regards to gout.

Alcohol can be a tough thing to give up, even if you are only a recreational drinker. Everyone has a different tolerance, and you should take a moment to think about yours. This is where keeping a food journal, as recommended in the chapter "Coping With

Gout" will help.

Your drinking may be what triggers your gout attack, but it might not be that all of your drinking is to blame. Think about the alcohol that you drink and go from there.

4) Dairy

Stick with low-fat options and options that are simply less rich. The Mayo Clinic recommends that you have less than 24 fluid ounces of dairy per day. Stick with skimmed milk and low-fat cheese. For example, Swiss cheese is relatively low in fat and can be safely eaten when you are worried about triggering an attack of gout.

When you are looking for something smooth and creamy, look for newer cheeses, which tend to be lower in fat, and consider adding a sprinkle of low-fat cheese to your sandwiches and your salad.

Move your milk consumption from whole or 2% milk to skimmed milk, and you will find that it is a lot easier to go through life without fear of a gout attack. Milk is one of the things that people with gout argue back and forth about. It is generally recommended by health sites that milk should be consumed carefully and only on rare occasions. However, there is a very high amount of anecdotal evidence that states that milk can even help during a gout attack. This is one of those things that is very dependent on who is being affected.

If you can cut milk out of your diet without much worry, sadness or trouble, it will certainly help you to lose weight. On the other hand, if milk is an important part of the way you eat, it might be worth experimenting with it to find out what your true tolerance is.

5) Refined Carbohydrates

Refined carbohydrates are broken down very quickly, providing your body with a fast sugar high. Some items that are very rich in refined carbohydrates include things like cake, sweets and white bread. When you eat too many refined carbohydrates, you do not leave enough space in your body for it to do the things that it needs to do. It can make it harder for your body to break down purines, and it can leave you feeling very tired and logy.

Take a moment to think about the refined carbohydrates in your life. They are often such a basic part of your life that you cannot separate them out. Be willing to take a moment to read the labels on the back of packages and to make sure that you are getting what you need.

6) Vegetables

It hardly seems fair, but the truth is that there is a list of vegetables that are high in purines. Not only should you go out of your way to avoid things like red meat and seafood, you should also think about some of the vegetables out there that are high in purines.

Brassicas like cauliflower and broccoli are fairly high in purines, as is asparagus, and spinach. You should also be careful with beans in general, though the worst offenders tend to be Lima beans, green beans, kidney beans and navy beans.

Some people have issues even with mild oatmeal, though other people seem to have no issues at all. As with anything else, the food that you can eat is a personal thing.

7) Great Foods for Gout

There is a lot to learn when it comes to figuring out the food causing gout in you. Learning what the causes of gout are and what foods to avoid if you have gout is an essential part of thriving with this condition, but you'll find that you also want to have some foods that you can eat without a problem. Happily enough, you will find that just as there are foods that will give you some serious problems, there are also foods that are going to make you feel a lot better.

For example, most poultry except for duck and goose is fine. Skip the pates and the dark meat on the turkey, but nearly everything you can do with a chicken breast is a good thing.

Black cherries are actually a fantastic way for you to reduce the amount of purines in your system. Some people eat them throughout the year, while other simply gorge on them when they think they are going to be having an attack. Check the Black Cherry Juice entry in the Great Gout Recipes chapter to learn more.

Whole-wheat items are going to be a great addition to your meal. Not only do they, on the whole, contain less refined carbohydrates than other starchy foods, they are also quite wonderful because they are also good for heart health. Whole-wheat items can be a little difficult to get used to when you are working on getting your treatment of gout under control, especially if you have been used to the standard white flour pastas and things like that.

The thing to remember is that you can learn to enjoy whole-wheat items for what they are, instead of being wistful for what they are replacing. As you start your purine diet, do not think that whole-wheat bread is something that is looking to replace white bread. It will simply not be as soft or as sweet. Instead, relish the nuttiness of the bread and appreciate it for its own merits.

The same goes for brown rice. Brown rice is chewier than white rice and takes longer to prepare, but the truth is that it does very well in a number of great dishes. Brown rice can be substituted for white rice even in things like sushi, and you can really learn to enjoy it on its own.

Besides the vegetables listed above, you are generally free to have as many fruits and vegetables as you like. Learn to make salads, soups and other veggie friendly dishes, and remember that you can find a way to enjoy them that is not simply related to wishing they were meat!

Be very careful around veggie burgers, however. Some of them are made with beans, and others are made with high soy content, and both of those things can trigger a gout attack if you are very sensitive. Make sure that you are checking the ingredients before you purchase them. Check the chapter "Great Gout Recipes" for a veggie burger made with lentils or rice.

You can have just about all the fruit juice that you like. If you are looking for a good way to get rid of soda in your diet, any gout diet PDF will tell you that juice is a great way to go. Orange juice and apple juice are both great ways to wake up, but as you go throughout your day, consider other juices, like guava, cranberry juice, and berry juices.

Chapter 8) Great Gout Recipes

Just because you have gout there is no reason for you to feel as if you have been denied everything delicious in the world. Gout is something that can and will limit your eating, but as you learn more about what food to avoid in gout diets and what can cause gout, you will realize that it is not as limited as you thought. As you put together the gout remedy report that works for you, you'll find that your gout diet treatment can actually look pretty tasty!

1) Brown Rice Sushi and Dipping Sauce

If you are someone who loves sushi, it will not escape you that some of the most famous fish for sushi, tuna and salmon, are considered high in purines and thus inappropriate for a gout-based diet. However, the truth remains that technically, sushi just refers to vinegar in rice, and there is no reason to skip the vinegary rice unless you want to!

Remember that brown rice is simply rice that still has the husks on it, and that for sushi, you should always choose brown short-grained rice. If you try to cook using long grain rice, your sushi will not stick together the way that it should.

Brown rice vegetarian sushi is a great dish to make when you want something a little luxurious, and all the extra equipment it takes is a bamboo mat designed for the purpose.

Ingredients

1 ½ cup cooked brown, short-grained rice

2-4 teaspoons of seasoned rice vinegar

2 sheets of nori

½ cucumber

¼ carrot

1 small avocado

6 tablespoons soy sauce

1-tablespoon sesame oil

1-teaspoon wasabi paste

¼ cup mirin

Allow your rice to cool to room temperature before you try to work with it.

Mix your seasoned rice vinegar into your cooked rice. The amount of vinegar that you want to put into the rice will vary from person to person. Some people like their sushi to only taste slightly of vinegar, while other people want a very intense flavor. Use your own discretion when making this decision, and keep who is eating in mind.

Lay one sheet of nori down on the bamboo mat.

Wet the nori very slightly with your fingers.

Spread a layer of rice on the nori, leaving the top ¾ inch and the bottom ¾ inch empty, but filling it out to either side.

Cut your cucumber and carrot into matchsticks

Peel your avocado and cut it into narrow thin slices.

Arrange the cucumber, the carrot, and the avocado in a row along the bottom edge of the rice. Do not overload this row of ingredients. If you put too many ingredients here, you are going to find that the sushi roll does not stay together. These are simply suggestions for ingredients to put into this sushi roll. Be creative and turn your sushi roll into real fusion cuisine. Leftover chicken fajita, pieces of pickled Japanese cabbage, and low fat cream cheese are all great choices for this recipe.

Roll the sushi from the bottom to the top, using your fingers to keep the roll tight.

Wet your fingers to seal the final free edge of nori to the rest of the roll. At this point, you should have a roll of sushi that looks like a log.

Pat the roll lightly with your fingers to make sure that it does not feel like it wants to come loose.

Repeat the process to create a second roll from your ingredients.

Use a very sharp knife to slice the sushi roll into coins that are about 1 inch thick. At this point, it is ready to eat as is, or you can continue on to make the dipping sauce as well.

Mix the soy sauce, sesame oil, wasabi paste and mirin together in a bowl. If you wish to do so, garnish it with very thinly sliced green onions. This is a great dip for sushi as well as other great Asian finger foods.

2) Applesauce Muffins

In many ways, a gout-friendly diet is one that is largely fat free. As with any change in diet, you will quickly start to miss the treats that you once had, but there are many other diet food options out there for you to try. When you are looking over diet meal plans and foods to avoid with gout, you may find that you are hungry for dessert. The best thing about applesauce muffins is that not only are they low in fat, they are intensely spicy, so you are not missing out on the flavor. As you look over gout foods to avoid, applesauce muffins will likely end up being one of your favorites dessert items!

Ingredients

1-cup flour

1½ to ¾ cup sugar, depending on how sweet you like your muffins

1-teaspoon cinnamon

½ teaspoon nutmeg

¼ teaspoon cloves

1-teaspoon baking powder

½ cup raisins

½ cup unsweetened applesauce

1/3 cup water

2/3 cup fat-free yogurt

2 eggs or 2 egg whites if you want to be very fat free

½ tsp vanilla extract

Preheat oven for 350 degrees Fahrenheit.

Mix the flour, sugar, cinnamon, nutmeg, cloves, baking powder, and raisins together in a large bowl.

Mix the applesauce, water, yogurt, eggs and vanilla extract together in another bowl, whipping until smooth.

Pour the wet ingredients into the dry ingredients.

Mix as little as possible while still mixing everything together thoroughly. The less you mix, the less you are working the gluten. If you overwork the batter, you will end up with muffins that still taste fine, but which will be more chewy and tough.

Pour the batter into a greased muffin tin. If you want to make sure that the recipe stays low in fat, use silicone muffin cups or cupcake wrappers to keep the calorie count down. If you want to add a slightly fancy touch to the muffins, make sure that you consider sprinkling some coarse sugar on top of the muffins right before they go into the oven.

Bake in the oven for about 18 minutes or until a toothpick inserted into the top of the cupcake comes out clean.

Serve warm or at room temperature.

3) Roast Root Vegetables

When you are looking to make a vegetarian main dish that is amazingly rich and flavorsome, consider roasting some root vegetables. Although this recipe is written for yams, beets and carrots, it can be adjusted to virtually any root vegetable at all.

Ingredients

2 yams

3 medium-sized beets

2-3 carrots

1 small yellow onion

2 tablespoons of olive oil

½ tablespoon garlic powder

¼ teaspoon salt

Light sour cream (optional)

Preheat your oven to 350 degrees Fahrenheit.

Peel your yams, beets, carrots and onion, and cut them into large chunks.

Throw the root vegetables into a pan.

Drizzle 2 tablespoons of olive oil over the vegetables.

Add salt and garlic powder to the vegetables.

Toss the root vegetables until everything is thoroughly coated.

Place the pan into the oven for 30 to 40 minutes or until the vegetables are cooked.

Plate immediately and serve with a dollop of light sour cream if you wish.

4) Vegetarian Lesco

As you look into gout causing foods, stop paying attention to what you cannot have and instead focus on what you can eat! Lesco is a Hungarian pepper stew, and in it's country of origin, it is served with sausage. The gout-friendly version of this dish is vegetarian, and it is quite delicious as a side dish or as a sandwich filling. Its fat comes from olive oil, which is thought by some to have some gout attack prevention qualities.

Ingredients:

2 tablespoons olive oil

1 small onion

3 yellow, orange or red peppers

1 banana pepper

2 cloves of garlic

1 tomato

Place 2 tablespoons of olive oil into a large pot and set it on the stove, heating it on medium.

Cut a small onion into thin strips, and drop them into the pot, stirring to coat the onion with the olive oil.

Cut 3 yellow, orange, or red peppers into strips and throw them into the pot as well. Do not use green peppers for this purpose, as they are too bitter.

Cut 1 banana pepper into thin rings, and throw it into the pot.

Mince 2 cloves of garlic and add it to the pot.

Dice 1 tomato, and add it to the pot.

Pour 1 8-oz can of tomato sauce into the pot.

Pour cups of water into the pot until all of the ingredients are covered.

Stir the ingredients together, and then turn the burner up to high.

Let the ingredients cook together for at least 1 hour, returning to stir occasionally and to add more water to the pot as necessary. Do not let the lesco boil dry.

Allow the lesco to cook until it is of a stew-like consistency, and then serve.

5) Turkey Burgers

If you are not actually a vegetarian, there is likely a chance that you have enjoyed a burger or two...or three or four! Burgers are great, but if you get them from the restaurant, they are full of red meat, which is a real problem if you are on a low-purine diet. This is where turkey burgers come to the rescue. A turkey burger is not made of red meat, but it can be delicious in its own right. Take a moment to consider how to make a truly delicious turkey burger.

Ingredients

1-pound ground turkey

Sprinkle of whole-wheat breadcrumbs or wet textured vegetable protein

¼ minced white onion

1 egg white

1 minced garlic clove

Salt and black pepper

Whole-wheat hamburger buns

Combine all of the ingredients together in a large bowl and mix them thoroughly. The amount of salt and pepper you add is up to you, but if you are feeling conservative, a light sprinkle of each will do.

Shape the mixture into patties with your hands. You can get 2 large patties or 4 small patties from this recipe.

Grill the turkey patties over a medium-high heat in a non-stick skillet until the turkey is cooked all the way through. You cannot serve turkey rare the way that you can with beef, so be certain that the patties are well done,

Place the patties on whole-wheat hamburger buns and add condiments as you please.

6) Lentil or Rice Burgers

When you want to enjoy something that is both healthy and flavorsome, consider lentil burgers. Lentil burgers give you plenty of nutrients without the fat and calorific load of meat burgers of any variety. This lentil burger is a fantastic choice when you are looking to cut calories and to make sure that you are still satisfied at the end of the meal. While you can of course top it with regular hamburger toppings, this burger goes quite well with salsa and a small amount of low-fat cheese.

While lentils are high in purines, some people report being able to eat them with no issues. If you are leery about lentils, consider replacing them with cooked rice in the recipe.

Ingredients

1-2 slices of whole-wheat bread

3 cups cooked red lentils or rice

3 eggs

½ teaspoon of salt

1-teaspoon garlic powder

1-tablespoon olive oil

Toast 1-2 slices of whole-wheat bread. When the bread pops, tear it into smallish breadcrumbs, and set it aside.

Mix your cooked red lentils, eggs, garlic powder, and salt very thoroughly, smashing them together until they are quite runny. If you have a food processor, this can make the process much easier. Do not worry if you still see whole lentils in the mixture as long as the texture is even.

Stir in the breadcrumbs.

Cover the bowl and leave it alone for ten minutes. This allows the mixture to come together a little more. You can add more breadcrumbs for a more sturdy texture if you prefer.

Split the mixture into 4 to 6 patties.

Pour 1 tablespoon of olive oil into a skillet and heat it over medium-low heat.

Lay the patties into the skillet and cover them with a lid, allowing them to cook for about 8 minutes.

Flip the patties and cook for another 5 to 7 minutes.

At this point, the patties are ready to be placed on whole wheat hamburger buns and served.

7) Sweet Potato Fries

When you are on a gout-friendly diet, you will discover that one thing that you might miss are potatoes. Potatoes are often considered an undesirable food for gout diets because they are full of empty calories, starch and sugar. However, the potato's relative, the sweet potato, is actually not only fine, but quite desirable! Sweet potatoes are full of vitamin A, they are full of anti-oxidants, and they provide a colorful splash to your diet. When you are looking for something to dip into ketchup and to accompany your gout-friendly burgers, consider what sweet potato fries can do for you.

Ingredients

3 large sweet potatoes

2 tablespoons olive oil

1 ½ teaspoon salt

½ teaspoon parsley

1 tablespoon of your favorite spice or spice mix, Cajun seasoning, mace, Bay seasoning, chipotle seasoning or allspice work well (Optional)

Preheat your oven to 400 degrees Fahrenheit

Peel your potatoes and cut them into wedges. If the wedges are very long, cut them in half.

Throw all of your ingredients into a large bowl and stir to cover the wedges in the oil and spice mixture.

Lay the wedges on a non-stick baking sheet or a baking sheet covered with aluminum foil in a single layer.

Place the baking sheet into the oven and bake for 30 minutes, removing the fries to turn them at the 15-minute mark.

Remove the fries from the oven and enjoy with ketchup, mustard, horseradish or your favorite condiment.

8) Black Cherry Juice

While you are cutting back on alcohol and probably on sodas as well, you may be really craving something sweet to drink. The answer can be found in black cherry juice. Black cherries have been shown to remove uric acid from the system, and if you make your own, you can ensure that there are no fillers or other harmful chemicals in them. Black cherry juice is on the expensive side to make yourself, but once you try it, you are not going to be satisfied with what you get at the store anymore! While you can use frozen black cherries for this purpose, fresh black cherries are much more delicious.

Cherry juice for gout is often included on a long list of gout medications, so when you are dealing with symptoms of gout in foot areas, you will find that this might be the perfect drink for you to make and then to freeze for later consumption. If you have never tried fresh, home-made cherry juice, now is the time to start. If you do not have the time or the inclination to make your own cherry juice, it is a good idea to consider black cherry supplements, which are available from most alternative health and vitamin stores.

Ingredients

2-3 cups pitted black cherries

2 cups of water

2 tablespoons Splenda or other low-fat sweetener (optional)

Combine all of the ingredients in a pan and bring to the boil, stirring occasionally.

When the cherries reach the boiling point, turn down the heat and simmer for another 10 minutes. Do not cover the cherries.

Mash the cherries until they are completely pulped. You can do this with a pestle, a large spatula or a potato masher.

Place a fine sieve over a bowl.

Pour the cherry mixture into the sieve.

Use a spoon to smash the cherries down until all of the liquid is drained into the bowl below.

Allow the cherry juice to cool completely in the refrigerator. You can keep the cherry juice for two to three days, or you can freeze it to save it for later.

Drink as is, or thin the solution with water.

9) Chicken Fajita

As you get away from a high purine diet and learn more about the causes of gout, you will find that you are eating a lot of chicken! The truth of the matter is that is that chicken does not have to be as dull as you were afraid of.

Chicken that is marinated, as in the case of these chicken fajitas, are quite tasty, and you'll find that as you realize what causes gout that it is possible to eat quite well. As you learn more about what the cause for gout is, you will discover more and more of these great recipes.

Ingredients

1½ to 2 pounds chicken breast

4 tablespoons olive oil, divided

2 tablespoons lime juice

1-teaspoon honey

½ teaspoon salt

½ teaspoon cumin

½ teaspoon chili

½ teaspoon paprika

1-4 cloves minced garlic

1 small onion

2 green peppers

Slice all of the chicken breast into strips and throw them into a re-sealable bag or a bowl with a lid.

Add the limejuice, 3 tablespoons of olive oil, the honey, all of the spices and the garlic to the chicken.

Seal the container and let it sit anywhere from 1 hour to overnight in the refrigerator. The longer you let it sit, the more flavorsome this recipe is.

Pour the marinated chicken into a skillet and cook on medium high until meat is lightly browned and cooked all the way through.

Remove the chicken from the pan and place it on a paper towel to drain.

Slice 1 small onion into strips as you get ready to start the meal.

Heat 1 teaspoon of olive oil in the same skillet. If you are very worried about fat consumption, skip the olive oil and simply cook the onion in the oil from the marinated chicken.

Brown the onion in the skillet, stirring regularly until the onion strips are soft.

Slice 2 green peppers into strips when you are ready to start cooking the meal.

Turn to low or medium low, and cook the green peppers and onions until they are soft.

Stir in the chicken, and mix until everything is equally warm.

Remove from heat and serve on brown rice, on whole-wheat tortillas or on whole-wheat bread.

10) Vegetarian Vegetable Soup

One of the unexpected things that might surprise you when you are looking at foods to avoid when you have gout is that you have to be careful with soup. Even soup that is low in fat is frequently made with chicken stock, and chicken stock is often cooked from bones and connective tissue, which are full of purines and high on the list of foods to avoid if you have gout. When it comes to gout, uric acid and the foods to avoid for arthritis in general are very high on the list of things for you to be thinking about. Check out foods to avoid gout, and learn more about how to cook well with this fantastic basic vegetable soup recipe.

This soup is a fantastic choice when you are looking at throwing something together for a cold day, and you'll find that as with a number of different soups, it gets better and better as you heat it up. To turn this simple soup into a light meal, consider adding a whole-wheat roll spread with some reduced fat butter.

Ingredients

1-tablespoon olive oil

1 small white onion

2 carrots

1 small zucchini

1 stalk of celery

1 large tomato

1-teaspoon salt

1-teaspoon oregano

1-teaspoon black pepper

3 16- ounce cans of vegetable broth

1 8-ounce can of tomato paste

Heat 1 tablespoon of olive oil in a large pot.

Slice 1 small white onion into strips, and brown gently over a medium heat.

Slice two peeled carrots into thin coins, and throw them into the pot.

Slice 1 small zucchini into thin coins, and throw them into the pot. For some visual variety, peel the zucchini in alternating stripes, letting the white of the zucchini's flesh contrast with the dark of the peel. This makes for a lovely contrast in the soup.

Cut 2 celery stalks into small pieces and throw the pieces in.

Dice 1 large tomato, and throw the pieces into the pot.

Add all of the spices, the broth and the tomato paste.

Add enough water to cover everything.

Bring to a light boil, and then turn down to a low simmer.

Cook until the ingredients are soft. This usually takes between 30 minutes to an hour, but you can cook to your taste. Some people really love a very mushy soup, while others like a little bit of toughness to their vegetables.

Serve hot with a slice of whole-wheat toast. Some people also throw a handful of whole-wheat pasta into the soup as it is cooking.

11) Simple Risotto

As you are struggling with the causes of gout and what not to eat if you have gout, you will find yourself craving simple, homey dishes that you can prepare with the ingredients you have to hand. When you are wondering what gout diet to do, take a moment to learn to cook risotto.

This classic French dish is often a little intimidating, but the truth is that it is quite easy, and thanks to the starch in short-grain rice, it is also quite rich without having the fat that often goes with a really tasty dish. Risotto takes time, but the end results are worth it. While you are struggling with your gout medication, learn to make risotto that will serve as an excellent comfort food and a great food for your entire family in general.

Ingredients

1-tablespoon olive oil

1 small white onion

1 cup of any short grain rice, though Arborio rice is the best for this purpose

4 cups of vegetable broth

Salt and pepper

Heat 1 tablespoon of olive oil in a large skillet.

Slice the small white onion into strips.

Sauté the onion in the skillet until it is brown and soft.

Turn the heat to medium-low

Add the raw rice to the skillet, stirring with a wooden spoon until every grain is covered with oil.

Heat the vegetable broth in another pot, and allow it to rise to a steady low simmer.

Add a ladle of the vegetable broth to the heating rice, stirring thoroughly so that the broth is completely absorbed.

Stir until you can no longer see any broth in the rice.

Add ladles of broth and stir them in until all of the broth has been absorbed. At this point, the rice will have released its starch, creating a texture that is very rich and creamy despite not having a bit of animal fat or dairy in it.

Serve hot, adding salt and pepper to suit individual tastes. Some people add a sprinkle of parsley over the top to add some color, while other people add a bit of low-fat Parmesan cheese.

12) Skordalia

When you are looking at what gout is and what causes it, and when you are busy concerning yourself with foods to avoid in gout and gout treatment foods, you might start craving something that feels a bit like junk food. With gout symptoms and causes and home remedies, gout is something that can seriously make you long for some easy chips and dip.

While a lot of dips are high on the list of gout foods to avoid, you will find that this Greek dip is perfect as a low-fat, low purine snack. Remember that potatoes can be a risky food for some people, but if you eat a smaller amount, you should be fine. Skordalia is a traditional Greek dish, and it can be used as a sandwich spread or a dip. It is strongly flavored and a perfect choice when you are looking for the perfect snack.

Ingredients

2 russet potatoes

8 cloves of garlic

½ cup olive oil

1-teaspoon salt

1-2 tablespoons of lemon juice

Peel and boil the russet potatoes until they are soft, and then set them aside.

Peel and mince the garlic. If you want a milder taste, simply crush the garlic very thoroughly.

Place the potatoes and garlic in a large bowl.

Add olive oil, salt and lemon juice.

Mash thoroughly with a potato masher until the skordalia is smooth. If you want the texture to be a little silkier, add some water.

Serve cool, with pita chips or with sliced vegetables.

13) Orange Sesame Chicken

Just because you are on a gout-friendly diet does not mean that you need to be in a situation where all of your foods are dull. Learning to cook with a worldwide flavor will quickly catch your interest, and as you learn what foods have uric acid and which gout treatment diet works well for you, you will quickly realize that it does not all have to be bland!

This orange-sesame dish comes from general Chinese-American cuisine, and it contains none of the foods that you have to avoid for gout. As you look into a low purine diet for gout and start looking at food to avoid, this is one recipe that is sure to get revisited time and time again.

<u>Ingredients</u>

2 tablespoons sesame oil, divided

1½-2 pounds chicken breast

3 cloves garlic

1 inch of fresh ginger

2 carrots

1-2 cups peas

¼ cup apple cider vinegar

¾ cup orange juice

2-3 tablespoons soy sauce

1-tablespoon sugar

1-tablespoon honey

1-tablespoons cornstarch

Heat 1 tablespoon of sesame oil on the frying pan on medium-high heat. Remember that a great trick for getting the most flavor out of your oil in stir-fry situations is to start with a cold pan, to warm it, and then to add room-temperature oil to it. Be careful of splatters if you do this!

Slice the chicken breast into strips.

Mince your garlic thoroughly.

Peel and mince your ginger thoroughly. If you are not sure that you want all that much ginger flavor in your chicken, you can simply cut the ginger into coins, and fish it out after the cooking is done.

Add the chicken breast, garlic and ginger to the pan, cooking until the chicken is thoroughly cooked and beginning to brown. Set the chicken aside on a plate.

Peel and slice your carrots into thin coins.

Pour 1 tablespoon of sesame oil into the pan and cook your carrots on a medium heat until they soften up.

Add the chicken back to the skillet.

Add peas to the skillet.

Pour orange juice, vinegar, soy sauce and cornstarch into a bowl and mix them until they are smooth.

Pour the sweet orange juice mixture over the contents of the skillet.

Cook for another 3 to 5 minutes over a medium heat. Stir with a paddle or wooden spoon to make sure that everything is coated thoroughly with the mixture.

Serve over brown rice or eat on its own. You can also sprinkle the top of the dish with toasted sesame seeds for visual variety.

14) Honey Balsamic Vinaigrette

As you start eating the gout diet, getting involved with gout treatment medications and learning about gout home remedies, you are going to get pretty tired of salads. People will start telling you that you can always have salad, but let's face it, if you were really in the mood for a juicy steak or a tuna sandwich, salad is a pretty poor substitute.

However, remember that salad on its own can be pretty awesome if you learn to make your own gout-safe dressings. When it comes to gout, what foods to avoid are important, but you also need to think about making the foods that you can eat even better. This honey balsamic vinaigrette is the perfect way to spice up a boring salad, and it definitely beats reaching for that bottle of ranch or French dressing one more time!

<u>Ingredients</u>

3 tablespoons balsamic vinegar

1½ tablespoons honey

¼ cup cold-pressed olive oil

¼ teaspoon coarse sea salt

¼ teaspoon crushed black pepper

Throw all of the ingredients together into a bowl.

Whisk thoroughly and serve on your favorite salads. This salad dressing is a great choice when you want to add a richer flavor to salads that are otherwise a little bit dull. For a little more zing, add more crushed black pepper to the mix.

Use sparingly as you add this to your salad. A little bit of this dressing goes a long way. If it is a little intense, you can thin it with water, though if you want something that is a little more intense, think about adding more honey or even some red pepper flakes.

15) Chai Tea

As you remove purine rich foods from your diet, and as you move forward towards finding the best home remedies for arthritis, you may find that you are in a spot where you miss sweet drinks. Some people are triggered by carbonated beverages, and when you are looking for something more interesting than water, you should think about chai tea.

Chai tea is an Indian recipe that uses spices and milk in black tea to create a warm and deliciously sweet drink. The ginger in the tea makes for an excellent gout remedy, and though it is not considered a standard uric acid treatment, it's a great beverage all on its own. Don't let yourself get so overwhelmed with low purine foods and learning about gout symptoms food that you end up denying yourself anything flavorsome!

<u>Ingredients</u>

2 cups of water

¼ cup honey

5 bags of black tea

1 cinnamon stick

4 whole cloves

¼ teaspoon of ginger

1/3 teaspoons ground cardamom

2 cups rice milk or almond milk

Boil 2 cups of water in a small pot.

Stir in all of the spices and the honey.

Remove the tags from the black tea bag, and toss them in as well.

Simmer everything for 5 minutes. You can simmer for 6 to 7 if you wish, but this makes for a very powerful black tea taste.

Remove the teabags from the liquid.

Add the rice milk or the almond milk. Both of these milks are great substitutes if you find that your gout attacks are sensitive to dairy.

Raise the temperature to high, and bring to the boil. Watch the pot, because boiling happens rather quickly.

Remove the pot from the stove.

Remove the cinnamon stick, and reuse it later if you wish to do so.

Serve as is, or, for a more professional presentation, simply strain it through a filter, a strainer or even cheesecloth.

16) Garlic Roasted in Balsamic Vinegar

When you are looking for a way to add savor to your meals but you don't want to pile on the fat or to mess with fat substitutes, you will find that vinegar and garlic are your friends. These are two flavors that are so closely related to meat and when they are combined you will find that they make an excellent garnish.

This recipe relies on garlic and balsamic vinegar coming together into a rich topping that goes well on pasta, on whole-wheat bread and on fish. It is an excellent choice when you feel as if you have been missing out on rich flavors.

Ingredients

4 heads of garlic

½ cup balsamic vinegar

½ cup olive oil

Separate and peel every single clove of garlic from the four heads, and cut off the tough ends. To make this process simpler, separate the individual cloves and place them between two bowls, closing them inside. Shake the two bowls vigorously, and most of the papery peel will just fall off.

Place the garlic cloves in a small saucepan, and cover them with the balsamic vinegar and the olive oil.

Turn the stove to medium-low.

Stir the garlic constantly for forty minutes or until the garlic yields to light pressure.

Remove the garlic from the stove and drain away the liquid. If you are feeling thrifty, you can use the liquid to fry something else or even to make a truly powerful pasta sauce.

Serve the balsamic vinegar infused garlic slightly warm or at room temperature. One great way to serve this item is to simply spread it on a slice of whole-wheat bread and then to sprinkle it with a low fat cheese.

17) Chicken Salad

When you are in a spot where you want to create a large batch of something for a picnic, or you just want something you can eat for a little while, chicken salad is a great choice. It makes an excellent side dish or sandwich filling, and once you make it, you can adjust the recipe as you see fit to make sure that you have something that you will always find tasty. This recipe is easily doubled or tripled or halved to create something that suits your needs for the day.

<u>Ingredients</u>

½ pound cooked chicken breast

½ cup grapes

¼ small red onion

1 stalk celery

2 tablespoons dried parsley

4 tablespoons low fat mayonnaise

3 tablespoons fat free Greek yogurt

1-tablespoon mustard

1-tablespoon apple cider vinegar

Salt and pepper

Shred the chicken breast finely using your fingers or a fork.

Dice the grapes, onion and celery.

Mix the chicken breast, grapes, onion and celery into a bowl.

Add the parsley, mayonnaise, yogurt, mustard, and apple cider vinegar.

Mix all of the ingredients thoroughly, until everything is covered.

Set aside in the refrigerator for at least an hour. If you leave it overnight, the flavors will blend more completely.

Add salt and pepper to taste. This recipe does particularly well on a whole-wheat roll.

18) Tomato Salsa

When you are eating a low fat and low purine diet, it is easy to forget that strong flavors are an option. However, if you are looking for something tangy and spicy, you'll find that a great tomato salsa can really liven things up. Use this tomato salsa as a topping for your favorite starches, to eat with pita chips or even as a delicious sandwich topping.

You may think that salsa is dull, but the truth is that until you have had it homemade, you don't know what you are missing!

Ingredients

3 tomatoes

1 small red onion

1 jalapeno

4-5 tablespoons lime juice

½ cup chopped cilantro

Dice your tomatoes roughly and place them in a glass bowl. A glass bowl is the best choice when you are preparing something as acidic as tomatoes, as it will not change the taste.

Mince your small red onion, and add it to the tomato.

Slit the jalapeno in half, remove the stem and rinse out the seeds.

Mince the jalapeno, and add it to the salsa. If you want a spicier salsa, add a Serrano pepper or a chili pepper to the mix.

Add ½ cup of chopped cilantro.

Mix thoroughly.

Cover the bowl, and refrigerate for at least an hour. The longer you let the bowl of salsa sit, the more the flavors will blend and the better it will become.

19) Pita Chips

After hearing all about the different things that you can use as dips and condiments, you may be feeling a little nervous about what you can use them with! Pita chips are a great choice when you are looking at finding something that is healthy and delicious. They are quick, and they can easily be added to any menu where you want something light and snack-like.

When you are thinking about making something special for a party, you can double this recipe easily. Basically, you simply need one tablespoon of oil for each pita that you decide to use. To cut back on the oil that is used, use a silicone brush to sweep it onto the pitas.

Ingredients

3 pitas

3 tablespoons of olive oil

Garlic powder

Preheat the oven to 375 degrees Fahrenheit.

Rub olive oil onto both sides of each pita.

Lay the pitas on baking sheets.

Use a pizza cutter to cut each pita into 8 triangular wedges.

Sprinkle the pita wedges with garlic powder. Add salt and pepper if desired.

Bake in the oven for 10 minutes or until crisp.

Remove from the oven and allow to cool slightly before consuming.

20) Grilled Chicken Sandwich

When you are looking at low fat recipes, you may be fairly startled to see how often chicken breast comes up. The truth is that chicken breast is a low fat protein that is relatively inoffensive as far as taste goes. That is why if you prepare chicken breast the way that you prepare your steak, you are going to be disappointed. Chicken breast, especially chicken breast that is purchased from a grocery store rather than a farmer or a farmer's market, is relatively tasteless.

Marinating your chicken breast gives it a fantastic flavor and it can make an excellent basis for a chicken sandwich with all of the trimmings. This is a deluxe chicken sandwich that is sure to make you savor every bite!

Ingredients

2 raw chicken breasts

2 tablespoons honey

1-tablespoon olive oil

2 tablespoons balsamic vinegar

2 cloves garlic

¼ teaspoon salt

Whole-wheat buns

Lettuce leaves

Tomato slices

Onion slices

Condiments

Throw the chicken breasts into a re-sealable plastic bag with the honey, the olive oil, and the balsamic vinegar.

Peel your garlic cloves and mince them up.

Add the garlic cloves to the bag.

Put the bag containing the chicken and the spices into the refrigerator and leave them overnight for the best taste. You can take them out in an hour or two, but the flavor will not be as bold.

Heat a pan on the stove until it is warm to the touch.

Remove the chicken breasts from the bag, and lay them on the pan.

Cook the chicken on high heat until both sides are seared.

Turn the heat down to medium low and cover until the chicken is thoroughly cooked. This may take between 5 and 10 minutes depending on your stove.

Toast your whole-wheat buns if desired.

Lay the chicken breasts on the buns.

Top with lettuce, tomato and onion slices, and add condiments as you wish. If you are trying to keep things low fat, use low-fat mayo and low-fat ketchup.

Index

Bilberry
Blueberry └ p.57
rapeseed
pineapple

CPSIA information can be obtained at www.ICGtesting.com
Printed in the USA
LVOW04s0025130415

434318LV00029B/1342/P